Obsessions, Rituals and Wasted Time

Days in the Life of Living with Obsessive
Compulsive Disorder, and Waiting for God to
Come to the Rescue

Donald E. Russell, Jr.

Publisher's Note
This work is based on the author's personal
experience of living with Obsessive Compulsive
Disorder.

"Almighty God, you know that we have no power in ourselves to help ourselves: Keep us both outwardly in our bodies and inwardly in our souls, that we may be defended from all adversities which may happen to the body, and from all evil thoughts which may assault and hurt the soul; through Jesus Christ our Lord, who lives and reigns with you and the Holy Spirit, one God, now and forever. Amen"

"Almighty God, the foundation of all wisdom, you know our necessities before we ask and our ignorance in asking: Have compassion on our weakness, and mercifully give us those things which for our unworthiness we dare not and for our blindness we cannot ask; through the worthiness of your Son Jesus Christ our Lord, who lives and reigns with you and the Holy Spirit, one God, now and forever. Amen."

– Collects from the *Episcopal Church's Book of Common Prayer*

Good Morning, World!

————————

Tap, tap, tap, tap.

"No, wait, the fan made that noise again."

"Okay, five finger taps on the mattress." Tap, tap, tap.

"Damn it!" Tap, tap, tap. "Sigh."

Tap, tap, tap, tap, tap. "There, I did it. It's done. Now let's get out of bed and start this day."

"Count to three, and throw the sheets off. Ready, one, two, three." Off they go, and I sit up with my feet flat on the floor.

"Are my feet pointing in the same direction?"

"Yes!" But were all of my fingers on the mattress while my feet were on the floor?

"No!" Back in bed, and under the covers I go.

"One, two, three!" Sheets off, sit up, feet down, with all my fingers flush on the mattress. My feet, however, are in slightly different directions, again. Taking a deep, exasperated breath, I get back in bed and under the covers.

"One, two three!" Sheets off, sit up, feet down, all fingers on the mattress, feet pointing in the same direction.

"YES!" Victory!

"If you get back in bed, you are going straight to hell."

"Make up the bed, now!" I have to make it up quickly so as to not get back under the covers. I also have to try turning off the thinking mechanism in my brain so as to not create a reason why I should get back in bed.

My wife turns off the water in the shower. "Get the pillows on the bed before the shower door opens." One, two, three... "Why does she insist on having so many pillows? Think of the money that went into all this fabric!"

The door to the shower opens. All the pillows come back off the bed and thrown onto the floor. After placing them back on the bed in the correct order, I say to myself, "Shoot eight birds at yourself and everything is cool."

Pulling at my hair in frustration, I think of my next-door neighbor rushing to get to the Pensacola Yacht Club marina on time, the guy across the street deciding which gray, cutoff wife-beater shirt he is going to wear to work in his yard, and of my other neighbor gearing up to play an early round of golf.

I, too, should be thinking about the day's awaiting challenges, but I am too busy opening and closing the bedroom door between the laughs on the radio. "There, I did it."

"Wait a minute. I am not so sure the door completely clicked in time. Didn't the lady chuckle there at the end of the comeback and not very funny joke on this ridiculous morning radio show? I better open and close the door again to be 100% sure."

"Oh, no!" Now they are breaking for a commercial, and

it is a car commercial with all the yelling and different echoing in deep and high-pitched voices. "Good credit, bad credit or no credit at all. Drag it in, tow it in, we will give you top dollar for any used car and you drive away without any down payment, zero percent financing and no payments until 2050."

I get back in bed and lay there on my stomach with a pillow over my head and my heart pounding. My senses are wide awake, but my body and common-sense judgment are in a loosing battle against the thinking mechanism in my head which has no cut-off switch, and it continues to create reasons for me to do things I against my will.

Even with all the repetitions performed this morning, the beginning of this day so far has not been a particularly bad one. Getting in and out of bed more than once is always a pain, but sometimes it takes me ten or fifteen times before correctly meeting the commands of my twisted mind.

Nevertheless, the awful process of the day is beginning, and my eyes, ears and sense of touch are revealing many obstacles and the games they present. Everything I see, hear or feel will play a vital role in determining winning or losing, health or disease, success or failure, life or death and good or evil. Even before the lights came on, my ears prompted my brain to play games with the songs blaring from the alarm-clock radio allowing me only to open my eyes between the disc jockey's obnoxious laughs, snorts and giggles on the awful morning show that only morons and idiots would find funny.

No matter that the sky is blue, and no matter the birds are singing, today is going to be another day of me fighting and living with my constant companion of the last 35 years – Obsessive Compulsive Disorder, commonly referred to as OCD.

Unscientifically, but relative to my experience, the five parts of OCD are:

- The Obsession – Overwhelming and unrealistic thoughts regarding an object, person, event or action.
- The Compulsion – The urge to perform an action (ritual) that has no purpose.
- The Ritual – The process by which one prevents a consequence.
- The Consequence – What may occur if a ritual is not completed.
- The Result – Anxiety and wasted time.

For example, I can become obsessed with a disease, and the consequence of that disease is it will kill all of mankind. The ritual I perform to prevent the consequence could be as simple as pinching myself four times, or as difficult as pinching myself 1,000 times.

My obsessions are constant, and I have spent about 80% of my waking hours performing rituals to prevent deadly or, otherwise, horrible consequences.

The entire world and everyone in it owes me a debt of gratitude for saving the world and saving each individual countless times. If it were not for my rituals, all would be sick or dead and the Earth as we know it would be gone.

I sincerely believed, during most of my time with this disorder, that I was the only one in the world who had it. I did not want to reveal to anyone my problem because I was afraid it was contagious, and infecting someone close to me with this sickness would leave me overcome with guilt and lead my friend surely to death.

For example, Jesus cast out many demons of the unclean during His ministry. He removed the demons from the person who was possessed and their health was restored. In the "Book of Mark," chapter five, Jesus removed the unclean spirit "Legion," who were many, and transferred them to pigs. The herd of two thousand then ran into the sea and drowned. I did not want to make a similar transfer of my disorder to anyone, not even a pig!

While trying to understand my own demon, I would ask, "Where is God, and why is He not helping me?" After waiting for years, He did not come to my assistance, so I went on performing ritual after ritual for a peace of mind that never came.

The Cure

Psychologists and psychiatrists have come up with a plan to fix all of this. It is called: Exposure and Response Prevention (ERP) – The method of intentionally putting yourself in the position of becoming obsessed with something, then denying the compulsion by refusing to complete a ritual to prevent the consequence. It is an exercise hoping to train the brain not to respond to obsessions. An extreme example would be making someone, who is so afraid of being dirty that they constantly wash their hands, walk around with a dead fish in their hands all day.

The subject is supposed to accept the fact they are dirty. Washing their hands will not prevent them from having germs because the dead fish will make their hands dirty all day long, anyway. Are you kidding, me? I would expect that to work for me like I would expect a wife to actually take a suggestion from her husband.

The problem of thinking my hands are dirty because of physical matter (in this case, a dead fish) is reality. A dead fish really would make my hands dirty, and even with OCD I can understand realities. It is the imaginary or invented thoughts making my hands dirty, so instead my mind needs to be dealt with, and not my hands.

Fortunately for me, my psychiatrist went the drug route. He started me out on 50 milligrams of Zoloft, and that did not scratch the surface. After the next session he moved me to 100 milligrams, and it made a little dent in the problem. After hearing more of my OCD stories, he prescribed 150 and then quickly 200. I figure anyone with OCD taking less than 150 milligrams of Zoloft a day is a lightweight.

As of the writing of this book, my prescription has not cured me of this disorder. The drugs do, however, keep my thoughts of doom and gloom to a minimum, and I hardly ever perform rituals anymore. My OCD will always be with me. I just have to beat it everyday with a hammer to make sure it stays below the limits of my sanity.

God has been my partner through all of this, and, like all partners, we have not always gotten along. I have loved Him and I have blamed Him, but in the end He came through with the hammer I needed to pound my problem into oblivion. As long as He continues to walk with me and provide to me His earthly remedies, I will survive this life in relative relaxation and happiness.

This book is my story of living with OCD, and it details my most common obsessions and most time-consuming rituals preventing unsatisfying or deadly consequences. The pain and suffering caused by this disorder clearly has taken a serious toll on my life. Although, there is a happy ending with me finally opening my eyes to God's gifts that were there all along. It is not a fairy tale with a happy ending; it is a horror story with a happy ending.

Those who live with OCD will understand it, hopefully get a laugh or two out of the proceeding chapters, and immediately seek help for this life-threatening disorder. Those who don't live with this disorder may find it an interesting story of someone suffering from what God can easily cure, if the victim does not wait for His help.

Rituals and Consequences

_____

The imagined consequence for not performing a ritual correctly could be, in the extreme, deadly. The pressure of completing rituals properly causes unimaginable stress and anxiety for a completely made-up consequence. Sometimes the rituals can't possibly be completed either physically or in a timely manner, so I always have a back-up plan.

The most common back-up plan for me is shooting ten birds at myself, saying "fuck you once, fuck you twice," or saying, "shit head" twice. These actions can solve most anything and have enabled me to save the world countless times. Should I be outside, doing cartwheels also helps immensely. I usually only use the back-up rituals should I realize the primary ritual is going to be impossible to complete. One time, however, I shot 1,000 birds at myself when I could never be sure I had shot 10 correctly. Even the foolproof rituals get out of hand sometimes.

The most common consequences for my not completing rituals are:

1. I would be possessed by the devil.
2. A US soldier would be killed.
3. The world would come to an end.
4. I would be killed.
5. The truck in front of me would explode.
6. My pet would die.
7. A family member would fall ill.
8. Auburn would lose to Alabama in football.
9. I would go to hell.
10. A lady would have breast cancer.

Usually, the only way to stop breast cancer, and this would be very embarrassing, would be staring at those very breasts for a number of required seconds. This was tough because that very person could very easily see me staring. But no matter, it had to be done, or this person may die of breast cancer. I would have the perfect excuse should I be caught checking out the cleavage or looking straight down this person's shirt: "Please don't slap me, because I have just saved you from the agony of chemotherapy and a mastectomy." They would surely understand.

OCD Pride

————————

My OCD is worse than anyone else's OCD. I can say that because no one can prove to me otherwise. My psychiatrist told me, once after I performed some of my rituals for him, that I was the perfect example of someone with OCD. Not knowing whether to take that as a compliment or an insult, I took it as a compliment.

Strange scene it was of me performing my rituals in front of my psychiatrist. I always pictured myself laying on a couch and explaining my troubles to a man taking notes while sitting in a leatherback chair. The office was nothing like I expected and had chairs facing each other over a desk with florescent lights buzzing overhead.

I am also an OCD snob and look down on others whom I consider crazy. For instance, I am not a constant hand washer. Some people wash their "germy" hands so much that they scrub them raw and bloody. Those people are insane!

I also feel very sorry for hand washers, because they are put in a very difficult situation when it comes to exiting a public bathroom. With today's technology, I can go to a bathroom without having to touch a flush handle, a soap dispenser, faucet or towel dispenser – those are all automatic with built-in sensors. The bathroom experience has almost become hands-free (except for the obvious). However, the one thing that must drive hand washers crazy is the exit door is never automatic, and the doorknob or handle is the most germ-infested object in any environment. Sometimes, though, no matter how creatively you try to open the door without touching the doorknob, it may become necessary to grab that nasty thing.

Should there be an automatic towel dispenser, I merely carry my used hand towel to the door and use it as a barrier while turning the knob or pulling the handle. I then toss the towel into the trashcan if it is in range, or carry it with me to the nearest receptacle.

Even though I don't consider myself to be an obsessive hand washer, I have come up with the following ways to "safely" open a bathroom door if, hanging on the wall, there is one of those worthless "environmentally friendly" hand blowers.

1. Should I be wearing a long sleeve shirt, I pull the cuff over my hand to turn the knob.
2. Should I be wearing a t-shirt, I use the shirttail.
3. If my shirt is tucked in, I stand on my tiptoes, and, with my hand in my pocket, grab the knob through my pants.
4. If the door is perhaps one at a gas station and does not

completely close, but leaves a crack, I wedge my foot in the gap and open it with my foot.

5. If the door opening does not have a crack, I grab the top of the door and make a crack for my foot to fit.

6. If the door is extremely heavy, and there is no other choice but to use the knob, I use my left hand and profusely wipe it on my pants afterwards.

7. If I am completely grossed out by everything in the bathroom, I won't even wash my hands (because by doing so I would be even filthier). I just hope someone else enters and opens the door wide enough so I can walk out without having had touched anything in there but myself.

The one thing about the bathroom situation I find puzzling is the evolution of automation. Wasn't the door automated before bathroom accessories? Then why is it the only hand operated apparatus in modern bathrooms that is not hands-free? I guess that is one of those questions that are answered upon our entrance to Heaven (along with who killed JFK, where is Jimmy Hoffa's body, who built Stonehenge, did OJ Simpson really do it…?)

Aside from considering myself to be mentally superior to hand washers and learning to live with manual bathroom doors, I have *earned* my position as one of the best and most accomplished Obsessive Compulsives. No one holds a candle to me, and I am greatly offended when someone claims to be or claims someone else to be, "so OCD."

The acronym OCD is being thrown around so much these days, it has never rightfully gained its stature as a serious mental condition. People say "Oh, he's/she's so OCD" because their closet is always straight, house and car are always clean, pencils are always sharpened, laundry is always done, desk is so organized...

With my level of OCD, hearing someone else say of these kinds of people, "Oh, he/she is so OCD" is like saying someone with a sprained ankle is, "so paraplegic."

The Mind (or the Brain)

When my mind began consuming my life with obsessions and rituals, I wondered how this could be happening. Why was my mind doing this to me, and why was God allowing this hell to become part of my life?

One of the differences between humans and other living creatures on earth is God gave humans a brain far superior to those of other animals (He also gave us opposing thumbs, but that is a subject for another book by someone else). Not taking away positive attributes of other animals, and not wanting to offend those who think dolphins are smarter than we are, but we are at the top of the food chain for a good reason. However, I believe ants have a better work ethic than we do, but sometimes their choice of anthill location comes into question.

During the 22 years my mind was requesting me to perform certain rituals to save the world, I eventually came to realize that the mind is a very powerful source capable of producing obstacles extremely difficult to overcome.

To realize the power of the mind, you only need to look

around to understand its incredible influence on our lives. Everything we have is because of our mind or somebody else's. (Thank you God for the "somebody else's," because my mind could only produce just above a 2.0 college GPA.)

Looking around my house, I see the influence of Thomas Edison, Alexander Graham Bell, John (the guy who invented the toilet), Steve Jobs, Bill Gates, Benjamin Franklin, Thomas Jefferson, George Washington Carver and the Wright Brothers (I have to look outside my window for that one).

Great men and women have come forward to do great things for countries and the world including George Washington, Winston Churchill, Captain James Cook, Helen Keller, the Rev. Martin Luther King, Jr., William Shakespeare, Franklin Roosevelt, Gandhi and Mother Theresa.

There are also the societies that influenced governments and infrastructure like the Greeks, Romans, Incas and Egyptians, and there were those who bestowed evil upon the world including Pol Pot, Hitler, Idi Amin, Mao Sedong, Joseph Stalin...

All of these people had incredible brainpower. Whether used for good or bad, the brains of these inventors, leaders, writers and dictators were either far superior to most others, or they were just used in ways other brains have not. The interesting point about dictators is they used people with little brainpower to carry out their atrocities, proving the theory of a great doctor that there are a lot more stupid people in the world than there are smart people.

Our minds dictate our lives in simple ways, opening up

new phases necessary for us to continue living a normal existence. There is no on/off switch for the brain, and it usually takes its time in transitioning our behavior.

For instance, we suddenly decide the following during the course of our lives:

- Ages 1-2 – Getting around by walking is easier than crawling.
- Ages 2-3 – Going to the bathroom in our pants is gross.
- Ages 6-8 – Paying attention when someone is talking is a good attribute.
- Ages 9-11 – Bathing everyday is a good idea.
- Ages 11-14 – The opposite sex really does not carry germs, but is quite attractive.
- Ages 18-24 – Education and having a job is not much fun, but learning and making money is necessary for success.
- Ages 25-30 – Our parents have always been smarter than we previously thought.
- Ages 25-35 – Marriage might be a good idea.
- Ages 25-35 – Having children would be fun.
- Ages 35-50 – Reading is a pleasure.
- Ages 35-50 – Working for money to save is smarter than working for money to spend.
- Ages 35-50 – Yard work is rewarding.
- Ages 55-70 – Working to live would have been better than living to work.

- Ages 75-85 – Wearing dark socks with shorts is okay for men, and panty hose with open-toed shoes is okay for women.
- Ages 85-100 – Falling asleep while someone is talking to you is acceptable.
- Ages 85-100 – Going to the bathroom in your pants is okay.
- Ages 85-100 – Death might not be such a bad thing.

The brain may also cause us to make stupid decisions including getting tattoos, drinking and driving, committing crimes, dropping out of school, wearing pajamas in public and throwing cigarette butts and chewing gum in urinals.

From a mental standpoint, the brain is an incredible source of power; it has the capability to completely overtake our ability to operate as our heart would rather us operate. Schizophrenia, insanity, insomnia, OCD, ADD, Dyslexia, Autism, Alzheimer's, Dementia, paranoia and Tourette Syndrome are just a few of many life-controlling disorders. During my fight with OCD, a small voice has always whispered to me to act against the obsessions created by my brain. This small voice was my heart, and it was always shouted down and drowned out by the enormous and thundering voice of my out-of-control brain.

Thomas Jefferson wrote one of the greatest analogies of the arguments between the mind and the heart in a love letter to Maria Cosway, a woman he met while he lived in Paris. In the letter, "My Head and My Heart," a conversation ensues between Jefferson's head and heart regarding the relationship between him and Mrs. Cosway. Throughout the letter, Jefferson's head and heart blame each other for the consequences of loving someone who could not possibly become his life-long companion, because Maria Cosway was married and her home was in Europe. Jefferson knows he will have to return to America. In the letter, the head speaks logically and the heart speaks with emotion. Jefferson writes a passage told by the heart to the head, "When nature assigned us the same habitation, she gave us over it a divided empire. To you she allotted the field of science, to me that of morals." The head says to the heart "Harsh therefore as the medicine may be, it is my office to administer it." Jefferson points out the guilt his heart feels when his head controls certain outcomes. That is precisely what happens in my case with OCD. The head wins every time.

Within my existence, my heart was always the weak participant in the conversation, and the guilt I felt was always for that little voice trying so hard to convince me to deny my brain's obsessions. My heart could in no way help me to overrule that incredible powerful source of energy that made so many men, women and societies so great, or so evil.

Wasted Time
is Forever Gone

_____

When I was in second grade, my teacher at LaGrange Academy used to stamp papers with little red faces to show our grades. We had not begun receiving letter grades, but only satisfactory or non-satisfactory marks. The little red stamps consisted of a smiley face, a frowning face and a sleepy face. I always got the sleepy face because I could never finish my assignments on time. There were always better things to do like play with my pencil, look around the room, stare at the floor, daydream of inventions to do my work for me, and watch the clock. The sleepy face, of course, meant I was wasting my time. As a second grader, though, I had plenty of time to waste.

As I grew older, time was not really a factor because there was always the night. No matter how much time I frittered away during the day, I could always stay up late to finish whatever homework was incomplete. If I did not get it done during the night, I could always get up early to complete my assignments before heading off to school.

In college, time was never a factor except for the fact I could not fit in all the fun within a twenty-four hour day. Attempting to fit in *all* the fun meant having to cram for exams and writing term papers in one night. If the clock moved a little too fast, skipping classes to catch up on other classes was a good strategy. Fitting in "bullshit" sessions with roommates, freezing over with water Playboy center folds on sidewalks during cold weather, playing intramural sports, attending fraternity parties, celebrating football victories, playing Frisbee football in classroom buildings, watching the "Breakfast Club" and "Revenge of the Nerds" over and over again and doing anything except getting an education is essential for an exciting college life. Who cares about time?

Once I graduated, the apocalypse arrived. I am the only person I know of who cried on graduation day. I had the perfect life, a great apartment, good friends and plenty of freedom, and I was about to leave it and move back home to my parents' house. I had no job, no girlfriend and no future.

The day of my graduation from Auburn University ended with me sleeping in my boyhood room in my twin bed. Where had all the time gone? My parents were older, my sister was living in Birmingham working for a publishing company, and I was a college graduate who was expected to do something with my degree.

Time suddenly became a factor because I could not bear to spend another minute in an environment and lifestyle that should have been a distant memory. I realized suddenly that I had lived nearly one-fifth of my life if I were to live until I was a hundred years old. When I was in second grade, I had only lived one twenty-fifth of my life, so staring around the room and not doing my assignments was of little consequence because I had plenty of life left to live.

When the fraction of life lived is getting larger, time goes by quicker. There are different theories as to why, but it just happens. When a senior in high school, second grade seemed a lifetime ago. When my 30th-year class reunion came around, the 20th-year reunion seemed like it was just last year. I guess when my 60th-year reunion roles around, my 50th will seem like it took place just last week. As we get older, time becomes a dwindling resource.

OCD does not have any mercy upon one's schedules. Obsessions pop up without notice, rituals take time to perform to prevent consequences, and performing an action that has no purpose is a complete waste of time. Since some of my days were spent performing rituals 80% of the time, I lost a huge chunk of what could have been productive hours. I spent a significant amount of time trying to prevent disasters that would never occur, change the outcome of events of which I had no control, cure illnesses in people that had not materialized, prevent myself and others of being possessed by evil spirits, and put unnecessary miles on my car revisiting possible accident sites imaginatively created in my mind.

My life, between the times I was 14-years old until the time I started taking Zoloft, has a big fat sleepy face stamped on it. It represents the time lost, and time I can never get back. I won't say it is like the time lost serving out a sentence in prison (I do not know what that is like and hopefully never will), but it was time served for an undeserved mental disorder. I have a hard time forgiving myself for not getting help earlier, because wasted time is forever gone.

Obsessions and Rituals Exposed

Getting caught having an obsession and performing a ritual is like being caught by your grandmother reading a "Playboy" magazine. First, you feel ashamed, then guilty, foolish, and finally you have trouble facing her at the dinner table. So, yes, I have been caught reading a "Playboy" by my grandmother. On two similar occasions, the need to fulfill my day with things I thought were meaningful cost me dearly. Once in Thailand, on a beautiful beach in the resort area of Phuket, a beautiful lady and I stayed at a wonderful resort with palm trees leaning over the water, mango stands on the beach and locals who offered cheap massages right outside the hotel rooms. While on the beach in mid-afternoon, she suggested we go back to the room for some privacy. Any man in his right mind would have said, "Okay!" Since I was not in my right mind, I said, "Let me swim out to the dive platform and back first." She informed me if I did that, then she may just settle for a mango instead. I said, "It will only take a minute." When I got back, she had already made a move to the fruit stand.

On another occasion, during a trip with my wife to Malaysia, an island just off the beach of the resort where we were staying tempted me to explore. At the time, I was exhausted and should have followed my wife back to our cabana to get out of the rain and relax for a while. But there was this island, and I had to get to it. I climbed onto a jetty and rock-hopped a few hundred feet until I slipped jamming my left leg between two rocks. Scraped up and humiliated, I headed back to the room. The humiliation was not because of not making it to the island, but that I had tried against my will. I only did it because of my obsession.

After returning to the cabana, I sat on a chair with my head between my knees crying and practically begged my wife to help me to relax on vacations and to not try to do everything. This Malaysian vacation was on the heels of a honeymoon where I made my wife miserable because of my obsessions to see and do everything. I ignored the fact that the real reason for the trip was to please her and to experience a romantic and relaxing vacation. I blew that one, too. I wish to God I could do my honeymoon over.

One very cold day in LaGrange, GA, my wife and I awoke to a dusting of snow on the ground. I did not have the right equipment for such a monumental event. Since the snow would melt in a couple of hours, and instead of enjoying time with my wife in the snow, I obsessed over the need to drive over to my parents' house to get my ski gloves and after-ski boots. Against my wife's advice (during an obsession, no advice is acceptable), I drove our only car towards my parents' house. I write *towards* the house, because, at about the halfway point, where a number of children were playing, the car slid out of control and slammed into a telephone pole. This accident was so embarrassing because it happened in front of a bunch of kids, in spite of my wife who told me to stay home, and because my parents had to loan us a car.

When I was growing up, my family would usually spend summer vacations in Pensacola, FL. When I turned 15, my father gladly gave me the keys to the car so he could rest easy while I drove the family back to LaGrange at the end of our vacation. At the time, Pensacola was home to the aircraft carrier, "The USS Lexington." Unfortunately, I could see it from the bridge crossing Pensacola Bay, albeit from five miles away. Whenever I crossed that bridge, I obsessed about having to look at it. This time was no different, even though I was behind the wheel.

My father, ever the observant one, noticed me looking over towards the carrier and not paying attention to the road. He told me to direct my eyes towards the direction I was going. I did for a few seconds, but then I had to look at the carrier, again. This time he said, "If you must look at the carrier, I will hold the wheel." What a way to build trust. Regardless of the chances of me possibly crashing the family into Pensacola Bay, or, even worse, looking like a fool to my father, I had to satisfy the obsession.

One of the worst "caught ya" incidents also took place on a vacation. My parents had just finished packing the car for the trip home when I announced I would run back in the house to make sure we didn't forget anything. The intentions were good, but when I got back in the house, I had to jump up and touch the skylight 20 times to prevent us from having a wreck on the way home. At about the number 13, I noticed my father standing in the doorway looking at me, and wandering what the hell I was doing. "What are you doing? We are in the car waiting on you!"

If only he knew that what I was doing had a direct impact on the safety of our upcoming journey. I was very upset after that incident, and all the way home I played obsession games trying to prove rituals were a farce. I would look at other cars and trucks on the roadway and obsess that they would explode if I did not perform a certain ritual. I would never perform the ritual, and the cars remained intact and never were consumed in an inferno.

Although I proved on that trip rituals had no correlation whatsoever to preventing consequences, my OCD had only just begun and was going to torture me for 23 years and grow worse year after year.

Beginning the Day with OCD

After finally getting out of bed in the morning, walking to the bathroom is an easy task. My body has suddenly realized it is time to pee, and nothing should get in the way of that morning priority. The bathroom is where "it" is all happening. Steam is moistening the ceiling, the hair dryer is blowing hot air and the hair iron is heating up. There is a small circle of reflection in the fogged up mirror in preparation for the application of make-up.

Thank goodness for three-gallon tank toilets. If these things were quick on the fill-up, I would be flushing them all day trying to make things right, but slow and steady make moving away from the toilet very easy. While walking away from the throne-room door and shutting it at the same time, I make sure my foot hits the floor at precisely the same time the latch hits the doorjamb. Perfect!

After saying good morning to my wife, she looks at me and mumbles something about fixing her breakfast. So out come the raisin bran and milk. I try to place the milk on the counter at the same time the refrigerator door closes, but miss. I open the refrigerator door again, place the milk back in, close the door and try again. The mission is successfully accomplished!

The next moment of my day is putting the flag up and retrieving the paper. Getting the flag to its holder in the front of the house is particularly hard. Our country is at war and if the procedure is not performed correctly, a soldier may loose his or her life in battle.

Upon exiting the house, my foot must land on the sidewalk at the same time the door latch hits the jamb. While stepping off the first step, I hold my foot up for as long as possible before letting it hit the ground. I almost fall and hurt myself, but, no matter, the procedure must be repeated so to do it correctly. I walk back into the house and repeat the procedure. The flag is in my left hand, so the door is closed with my right hand, and I move forward off my left foot and take a step toward the sidewalk. I let go of the doorknob as it begins to close on its own. My right foot swings past my left leg. The door is not closing fast enough, so I have to delay putting my right foot down. My body moves down the step too fast and my right foot comes down on the sidewalk…click goes the door. On the fifth try, I get it right and hope to God none of the neighbors saw me.

I round the corner of the sidewalk to place the flag in its holder and twist it until it is perfect, and then head to get the paper. At the tube, I reach in to get the paper, grab it and pull it out and begin walking toward the house. My foot, however, was in the road and on the driveway at the same time, and that should not have been. I place the paper back in the tube, take three steps back and retrieve it again with both my feet completely in the street. I then run to the front door and try not to notice anything that might make me do something I do not want to do…like stepping on a crack in the sidewalk.

"Did I step on a crack? Yes, I think I did." I go back to the driveway and have a meeting with myself to make sure I only mean the expansion cracks and not the hairline cracks appearing over time. When the meeting is adjourned, I understand I am only speaking of the expansion cracks and run back to the front door making sure no cracks are stepped on.

Once back inside, I open the paper, and a whole world of new games lay before me. I read in the same order everyday, starting with the front page. If having to read about a soldier or soldiers killed in battle in Iraq or Afghanistan, the story will be far into the past once the end of the paper is reached. The thing I really hate is if a story continues on an inside page. The last paragraph on the front page and the first paragraph on the inside page must be read twice to insure it is the same article. If I were I normal, I would quit reading the article because the remaining part of the story could not be that meaningful if it is not included on the front page.

The life section is not very important to me but it must be read and the less important the more difficult. The paragraph about Liz Taylor is really long, and I must read it without blinking. "Go, fast, hurry and you are almost there. The last line is near, I can make it" – blink.

Back to the top I go. "Quicker this time, only a few words to go, my eyes are getting dry and starting to sting. The last line, the last word." – blink.

"Did I make it? Mission accomplished? It was close. I better do it again just to make sure."

The comics should be enjoyable and I must always read the "Peanuts." I hate "Dennis the Menace," but if even just part of it catches my eye, I have to read it. The same rule applies for "Garfield," "Jump Start," "Dilbert" and "Snuffy Smith." If it's to save the world, I will read them. The world owes me - all the countries and all of the people. If it were not for me, the world would surely have come to an end.

The hair dryer just went off in the bathroom, and I hear cussing because my wife makes the morning claim she is fat and has nothing to wear. She has more clothes than I would want and certainly we could retire on the money spent on her clothes and shoes. She is also not fat; she is beautiful. However, all of the noise and slamming of objects is my cue to fix her lunch.

I don't do it because of obsessions or that anyone may die or the world may come to an end. I do it because it will save me five dollars and because she might put me on a pedestal for preparing it. As time has gone by through the years, though, I find it only saves me five dollars.

Fixing her lunch also increases the number of duties in my score column. I don't want her to say she does more for me than I do for her since some marriages turn into a game of keeping score with how much one does for the other. But in my case, it is not what I do but what I don't do. In other words, after a full-day's work in the yard cutting the grass, trimming the hedges, weed eating, pruning the trees and edging the sidewalk, I would be greeted at the door with, "I just sent you out this morning only to take out the garbage and sweep the front porch. What the hell have you been doing all day?" With OCD, you can easily get distracted.

My wife's car is loaded with her workbag and lunch, and she leaves complaining she is late again. Hoping she will leave me with a positive, uplifting expression, she only asks if her Diet Coke is in the cup holder, and off she goes. I am left extremely depressed. The garage door shuts behind me as my foot hits the floor in perfect time.

Back to the newspaper and a fresh bowl of cereal, I eat quickly and try to read all the news. As soon as the last spoon-full is eaten, the bowl is immediately rinsed. No world is worth saving if a ritual requires me taking one more bite of raisin bran after it has reached the point of ultimate sogginess and disgusting taste. All of the raisins, however, are eaten. The paper is finally read and put away. Fortunately, there were no news stories of tragedy where I may hold myself responsible.

The shower awaits, and not an exciting one, because I have taken a shower the exact same way for the past 22 years: water on, step in, wash hair, rinse, wash hair again, rinse, soap up arms, torso, legs, underarms, face, rinse face, legs, arms, shoulders (left, right) and under arms (left first, then right).

"Did I rinse my underarms? Rinse them again!" Shoulders, then underarms.

"Damn it! I did not do my shoulders, did I?" Do them again, and this time in the right order.

Shoulders, underarms. "Done. Perfect."

The water is cut off quickly before I have a chance to renege on my accomplishments. "Shoot two birds at yourself or say 'shit head' twice."

"Shit head once, shit head twice."

"Did it! Everything is cool." The towel comes off the rack and I dry my face first, torso, legs, arms and face. The towel is then flipped over my head and onto my back. I shake my head like a dog, and this is done without exception, even on days when I have a hangover or a headache and shaking it will only make me feel worse. Never mind, though; it must be done. If I do not stick to my routine, Auburn may not beat Alabama next year, and I would hate for them to lose on account of me not shaking my head.

Getting dressed is fairly easy because my work is quite casual and khaki pants and golf shirts are the norm. Sometimes, however, my pants need ironing and this morning is no exception. Out come the ironing board and iron. My wife loves doing my laundry, but she would never do my ironing. Once finished, I unplug the iron and make sure it is unplugged. I would not want the house to burn down, and have my wife come home in tears with all our stuff gone and the cat dead.

I must get to work and finally do. Work is good because it is real, and sometimes I hope for a crisis so reality will have to be dealt with and not so much fantasy. It is unfathomable to wish something would go wrong at work costing me time and money, but working to solve a real problem takes my mind off of having to save the world should my feet be pointing in different directions. Solving real problems is also sometimes a lot less stressful than completing rituals to prevent an imaginary consequence.

The morning routine is fairly common as any home-office activity would be. Turning on the computer is the official start to the day and Excel spreadsheets help me to plan the sales calls to be made throughout the afternoon.

The combination of raisin bran and looking at a computer work like a laxative. Off to the bathroom I go, and there is no OCD to stop this rush. I reach for the roll of toilet paper of which there is none. "I just put a full roll on yesterday morning! How could this be?"

The answer being one of the goals of some women when they awaken in the morning is to go through an entire roll of toilet paper before the day's end. Some also seem to like using, to the extreme, the aerosol can (hair spray, air freshener) and the squirt bottle (contact lens solution, dishwashing detergent and toothpaste). Should our toothpaste tubes be able to press charges for abuse, I am sure they would. One more related product to toilet paper would be the paper towel. What would take me a half a sheet to clean up a spill would take some women ten. There is just some kind of feminine thrill they get from yanking, ripping and wadding up. (Kind of like what they do to men's hearts in high school and college.)

Back to my problem of lack of toilet paper, I waddle to the cabinet, which I find empty, and then waddle to the other bathroom and thankfully find some there. Job well done. Now back to work.

OCD is not a factor in my hour of preparedness before I hit the road to make my sales calls, but it does kick in fully as I prepare myself to leave the house. With all of my work things gathered including a black notebook, white contract book, gray collateral crate, appointment diary, cell phone and wallet in my arms, I make my way to the car. I successfully place the objects into my car and make my way back into the house to get my lunch and bottle of water. "Did the cat get out while the door was open to the garage?" I call for my cat once inside, "Bugsy! Bugsy!" No answer. Not that I was really expecting one. I look in his usual places and find him in the towel basket. "Good."

I pet him, but did not get both ears. I pet him again and this time got both ears, but he swiped at me. I pet him again, and this time he drew blood with his sharp claws. One more time, and he missed me. He is not the kind of cat who likes to be pet more than once, and he is probably the only one who senses my OCD insincerity and thus knows my petting of him is not genuine after the initial act of affection.

I wash my hands and put some alcohol on the scratches, grab my lunch and head out to the car. While sitting in the driver's seat, I pull down the checklist taped to my visor and check off my work-related items: black notebook, white contract book, gray collateral crate, appointment diary, cell phone and wallet. "All there. Ready to go! Wait! Did the cat get out when I came back out to the car with my lunch?" Better go check the towel basket to make sure he is still there.

He is not where he was, and I know in my heart he did not get out. I must find him because if he gets run over by a car, it will be my fault. I find him in the guestroom sitting on the bed giving me that puzzled look he always does when he thinks he is being stalked. I pet him successfully and tell him that I love him and will see him tonight.

Once back out to the car, my mind goes back to the iron and the ironing board and of the house burning down. I go back into the house and make sure the iron is unplugged. For safety sake, I put it on the metal top of the dryer and face it away from where the cat may jump up and burn himself. I fold up the ironing board just to make sure I will not be able to picture the iron burning up the fabric on the ironing board. After placing it in the hallway closet, I close the door and ensure it latches so the ironing board can't escape.

Since, once again, the cat may have gotten out without me knowing it, I search for him again and find him on his kitty condo. I say goodbye again and tell him I love him. It may be the last time I see him, and I want him to know I love him.

I finally get to my car, again, and open the garage door and back out. I watch the garage door close, and drive out of the driveway. Halfway down the block I question whether the garage door closed. If it did not, an intruder could get through the unlocked garage door, steal the silver, or, worse yet, abuse my cat and then my wife when she gets home. My heart begins to pound and my mind forces me to turn my car around and go check the garage door. I get back to the house, and it is definitely closed. "Wait a minute. It did not close on a small animal, did it?"

I have read that if a garage door is not adjusted properly, it could crush a small animal that may have been trying to get in or out of a garage. Driving all the way back up the driveway and seeing the length of the garage door next to the concrete assures me everything is okay. I hate the thought of one of God's little creatures struggling under the weight of that door all day.

Finally, I head out of the driveway and leave my house behind, but I am dreading the commute ahead. I live in Gulf Breeze, Florida, but work in Destin, and that means my commute takes me down Hwy. 98, commonly referred to by most people who drive it as "Bloody 98." The name is attributed to the highway because of the many wrecks caused by drunk drivers, sleepyheads, speeders, stoplight and stop sign runners, the hundreds of driveways and country roads feeding into the main thoroughfare, school buses, school zones (what government official thought it was a good idea to put a school zone on a federal highway?), mail carriers, garbage trucks, short turn lanes, non existent turn lanes and careless cell-phone users. The one thing that could make it bloodier than it already is would be a driver performing rituals to prevent made-up consequences.

An automobile has so many things to distract from its purpose. The only thing an automobile is supposed to do is get someone from point A to point B. Somewhere in time, many other things were added to the automobile to detract from its original purpose. It has become a place for congregating, debating and laughing, an office, a powder room, a place to shave, dressing room and bedroom, a phone booth, concert hall and movie theater. It is also a moving piece of art, noisemaker and small-animal killer.

I watch some cars go by and wish I had the money in savings some people have put into their cars: amplified stereos, hydraulic lifts, enlarged engines, navigation systems, multicolored paint jobs, spinning hubcaps, thin tires and wide mag wheels, neon undercarriage lights, spoilers, air dams, PA systems, light covers, tinted windows, curb feelers, tachometers, roll bars, hunting lights, glass packed mufflers and a bunch of other crap you could either steal or purchase from an auto-detail store.

My cars have always been simple with no added accessories but plenty of distractions. There are so many things to play with including knobs, buttons, compartments, cup holders, electric windows, headlight flashers, air vents, mirrors, visors, the horn, windshield wipers and pedals. With all of this to play with, who has time to pay attention to the road?

The steering wheel is one of my favorite toys in the car. That is a good thing too, because while driving it is an important instrument to hold on to. With the steering wheel, I like to use the little reflectors in the middle of the road as an obstacle course. When passing a car, I try to either miss them all together, or try to hit one with only one or two tires. Drivers I have already passed probably wonder why I keep moving from lane to lane once the passing sequence has already been completed. Little do they know, I am trying to "get it right."

The Commute to Work

———————

Most of what I do regarding OCD is not so life threatening to other people until I get on the road. Sadly, defensive driving from other drivers probably won't help them predict what I may do behind the wheel when something as small as a speck on my windshield could play a role in saving the world.

On the road, there are so many games to play with highway features normal people take for granted. When engineers and laborers created a system of roads their legislatures so proudly under budgeted for, they had no idea they were creating a playground for a person with OCD.

Time conscious drivers are easily excited at the thought of making it through traffic light after traffic light. Excitement builds as a green traffic light is approached, and the closer the driver gets the more anxious the moment becomes. Getting through the green light is a victory. Otherwise, watching it turn yellow and then red forces a stop, which is a loss. The routine is something along the lines as, "Okay, here we go at a steady 55 mph and should I make it through this light, I will be at my destination on time."

Looking ahead at the road, all seems clear and the light is still green as I approach to within 500 ft. Now I am within 400 ft. and it is still green. "This one is going to be easy." 300 feet to go, and I declare, "I am going through it." 125 ft. between me and the light, and it turns yellow.

"SHIT!" I hit the brakes, and all my stuff that was in the front seat is now on the floorboard. My heart rate subsides and my hand hits the steering wheel. "Damn it."

I think to myself, "What the hell is this traffic light doing way out here in the middle of nowhere letting one car cross the highway from a worthless little side street?" Then I think of local city council meetings and someone complaining they can never cross this section of road without fear. Then a request is sent to the local, state and federal government for there to be a light right there to stop the whole of civilization on a federal highway to let some idiot from a little feeder road cross without stress. I guess you have to give it up to the politicians, because government only does two things well when it comes to roads: building them and then screwing them up by throwing up a bunch of traffic lights.

Bound and determined not to get stopped by the next light, I decide to blast through its yellow light. It turns red a little before passing underneath, but I made it, and my build-up of making it through did not come crashing down. "Did I hear a tire squeal as I went through? I think I did."

"No, it was not a tire squeal. It must have been something else. Was it a scream, did someone scream? Did I cause an accident? Did someone get killed?"

I look back in my rearview mirror. Everything looks okay. Traffic seems to be moving, although someone could be in a ditch or behind a tree. "I did not cause an accident. Don't be stupid. Everything is cool."

My palms are a little sweaty and my anxiety high a few miles down the road, and I continue to wonder if someone is in a ditch all bloody, and no one has noticed the broken vehicle on the side of the road. "I DID NOT CAUSE A WRECK," I scream at myself. "Don't be stupid. Everything is cool."

Upon reaching the next median cut, I think about turning around to go back and check to make sure all is okay. I hit my turn signal and slow down, then turn it off and hit the gas to return to normal speed. "I did not cause an accident, so let's just move on." I try focusing my attention to a song on the radio, but I see an ambulance coming toward me from the other lane with sirens blaring and lights flashing. My heart beats faster and words come from my mouth yelling at me to keep going. "That ambulance could not possibly be going the fifteen miles back to an accident I might have caused. If there had been an accident, it would not be this ambulance that was called. This one is obviously going to some other emergency that is much closer."

Before I know it, I am banging the steering wheel and cursing myself as I am now following the ambulance back to where I ran that yellow light. I try to relax once cooling off, because I know, in my heart, this is not a worthy trip back. The ambulance is still in my sights about a mile or so ahead, and I see it turn off to a side road away from the highway and away from my imaginary wreck. "Everything is cool."

My feet never hit the brakes nor do my hands hit the turn signal for the next median cut to make my U-turn back towards my destination; nope, I continue heading toward that traffic light to make sure there is no wreck. I have to, because someone is injured or dead, and I am responsible.

As I approach the light, traffic is moving swiftly through the intersection, no wrecks or injured people anywhere, and all is normal. However, I better keep going to the next light because of not being sure it wasn't the previous light where I heard the squeal. "No, no, no, it was this one. Damn it!"

My heart races, and I bang the steering wheel and proceed on down to the next light knowing damn well I am proceeding too far. I approach the light, and all is normal. I do a U-turn and head back the other way toward the light where I am sure I might have caused an accident. Within 250 feet it turns yellow, and I hit the brakes and stop just as it turns red. I have stopped, and it is just what I should have done before. All that wasted time. There is no wreck and no bloody pedestrian, and I knew it all along, I just had to prove it to myself. "Everything is cool, you idiot."

"Hey, I didn't cause an accident back there where I made that U-turn did I?" Hit your knee four times and everything is cool.

As I continue on my journey, a speck on my windshield has come into view. It could be the remnants of a smashed bug or bird doo. The speck on the windshield is only one if looked at directly, but two if looking past it on the road ahead. The same thing goes with any object in the foreground of a distant view. If you look at something beyond your index finger, your finger will appear as two. Focus on your finger, and you only have one, but that in the distance is now two. With OCD, you never miss anything.

The speck is positioned a little to the left of my direct view of the road, so I have to lean slightly to complete my next ritual: ten center stripes must past between the two specks before I can look up into the direction I am driving or civilization is doomed. Ok, one, two, three, four, five, six, seven – I have to look up.

One, two, three, four, five, six, seven, eight – almost there. One, two, three, four, five, look up…the car ahead of me is braking. No, it's just changing lanes. One, two, three, four, five, six, seven, eight, nine, ten! There, it's done, and everything is cool.

"Did I count nine, or did I skip it? I think I skipped it." One, two, three, four, five, six, seven. "Damn it, the middle line was outside one of the specks."

One, two, three, four. "Oh, no, I missed, again!" One, two, three, four, five, six, seven – I have to look up, a traffic light is just ahead. This is so stupid. Pop your thumb twice and everything is cool. "There, good."

I turn on the windshield washer hoping the dot will go away.

"Quick, read the top line on that billboard before the wiper passes over it. Try again. Try it on the next billboard. Try again. Floor the gas pedal twice, and everything is cool."

What the hell was all that for? There was not even a consequence for not completing a ritual. I spend half my day performing rituals that will not even result in preventing negative consequences. What a waste of time!

The windshield wipers add a whole new dimension to the game when there is something stuck under them, like a piece of pine straw. Trying to time the arrival of the straw as it moves with the wiper across the windshield is sometimes difficult when it is raining, and I am traveling at 55 mph. Eventually though, my timing is perfect and I yank the pine straw from underneath the wiper. The game is even more challenging when the pine straw is out of reach, and I not only have to time the arrival of the wiper, but lift it ever so slightly so to free the straw from the blade.

As the road stretches in front of me, the most dangerous of all rituals takes place. My eyes are to remain closed until I count to 10, or someone close to me will be kidnapped and abused. Counting up to seven or eight was common, but I could rarely, if ever, get to 10. One thing is for certain, though, an OCD driver is worse than a drunk driver. I could have so easily killed someone many times.

Riding my Bike

As a child riding my bicycle, I had similar obsessions. Some of them caused injury and pain, and others were just a pain.

Receiving my first road-worthy bicycle was like getting my driver's license. I was free to go just about anywhere had there been the time. However, similar to driving a car, I had to look where I was going, and with OCD, that was never quite so easy.

One evening, before my parents were going out, I decided to take the ol' JC Penny three-speed out for a spin. The bike had a pretty mustard-yellow colored frame, chrome handlebars, black lettering and a black seat. While heading down Ivydale Road, a red, James Bond looking car (probably just a Mazda RX-7) was heading towards me in the opposite direction. I saw it and thought it was really cool. Then came the obsession, and I could not stop looking at it. What the consequence of not completing the ritual of staring at this car was, I have no recollection. However, I do remember the consequence of the obsession: the front wheel colliding with the curb, a handle bar digging into my rib cage, my elbow striking the pavement, my legs twisting like bread-ties around the bicycle frame and the driver of the really cool car performing some kind of resuscitation procedure upon my scraped up body. I remember him lifting me by the waist of my jeans. Maybe he was trying to shake the humiliation out of me, but it did not work.

Another thing I used to have to do was pass over a rock without hitting it, but making it pass between my two wheels. Should I have missed, or hit the rock with one of my tires, I would have to turn around and make another attempt. In doing so, I would lose speed and time and be late to wherever I was going. The danger in performing this action lies in the quick action of jerking the handlebars back to a position making it possible for the rock to pass between the wheels. The possible result is overcorrecting the turn and flying over the handlebars.

On one such occasion, after completing a descent down a lengthy hill, an obsession overcame me, and I overcorrected a turn. I landed bruised and bloodied about 20 feet from what used to be my bike. The front wheel looked like a pretzel, the forks were all twisted and my beautiful handlebars scratched up. After asking a lady who was working in a nearby yard if I could use her phone, she looked at me as if I were going to take her into her house and beat and rob her. I don't know if she was shocked at my appearance, or thought I was a walking corpse.

My mother did come pick me up and was shocked to see me in one piece after seeing my bike. Again, I do not remember *the* consequence of not completing the ritual of overcorrecting, but I do remember *the* consequence: my mother bought me a bicycle helmet. The horror of having to wear that frightened me more than the possibility of having another accident.

Sales Calls

My profession is publishing tourist magazines in Northwest Florida. I stress "northwest" because we are different from the other part of Florida as we are mostly redneck conservatives who are not even considered when national elections or vacations for the rich and famous are considered. Our senators and governors are never from this area, and Democrats pretty much write us off as areas to politic or even promote. People only realize we are part of Florida during a good hurricane, but we did make a name for ourselves when we single handedly swayed the 2000 presidential election.

In order for me to publish magazines, I have to meet with people face to face and attempt to sell ads. Realistically, I am a door-to-door or an outdoor salesman. Being a salesperson requires social graces, speaking, listening skills, eye contact and body language. Those requirements sound like pressure enough when trying to take another person's money and put it into my back pocket. Politicians can pass laws in order to legally steal other people's money, but I have to do it honestly.

I possess the requirements to make a sale, but the neat thing is I could perform 100 or so rituals while I made a sale! The most common game would be darting my eyes around the face from feature to feature. While making my sales pitch, a game would begin involving darting my eyes from the customer's left eye, to the right eye, to the nose, to the mouth and back to the left eye. If a mole were in view, I would throw that in the sequence, too.

The imagined consequences could be any of the aforementioned, but the real consequence was if they thought me too weird to buy from. If the eye wandering was not enough, I would tap my pencil on the table, rotate my thumb under the table, shoot birds at myself, or dig my nails into my hands causing much pain. But through all of this, I could negotiate prices, design a thumbnail ad, and write up a product description. Sometimes it seemed as if the customer knew I was not quite right causing me to become embarrassed, and I could feel my face turn red. Nevertheless, I remain successful and good at what I do.

As written above, self-inflicting pain is also a ritual. When many other methods were exhausted in attempting to save the world, self-induced pain would often solve the problem. Sometimes, I wished physical pain would encroach on my being, so to take the place of the imaginary crises I had otherwise created. The most common forms of torture would include digging my fingernails into my skin, pulling my hair or rotating my thumb on its socket until it was sore. Punching the steering wheel was also very common, but I had to be in the car to do that.

One of the physical byproducts of my OCD is a grimace on my face. It may be mistaken as a smile, but it sticks sometimes for a while and takes place usually when there is nothing to smile about. People used to ask my sister why I always had that funny looking grin on my face.

Someone in college wanted to nickname me "Smiley," but it was not until years later I understood why. While driving down the road between sales calls, I would suddenly feel myself doing it, and would look up into the rearview mirror to see just how stupid I looked. Pretty stupid, and no telling how many times I may have done that in front of customers while at the same moment digging my fingernails into an unclothed area of skin.

One time, while stopped at a traffic light, a group of black men in the back of a pick-up truck were laughing and smiling, and pointing and waving my way. Having no idea how I was amusing them, I looked at myself in the mirror and there was that grimace. I tried to naturally smile back at the good-natured men, but my embarrassment was too great.

The grimace was the only symptom of my OCD that showed to those around me. I was so good at hiding all the other stuff, no one ever noticed. When someone asked about my odd smile, I would just shake my head and pretend not to know what they were talking about.

I do still make that odd smile, guessing it is something my Zoloft will not make go away. It was not the outward appearance of my being, though, that made my life so miserable, but the thoughts within. I can live with the occasional dumb look, but not with a bombardment of obsessive thoughts, and Zoloft has been affective in holding those inward afflictions to a minimum.

Proofreading

The grimace certainly comes into play a lot when proofreading my publications. Sometimes so much, I am afraid my face is going to be stuck in that position. OCD consequences certainly come in different forms and most commonly is a made-up consequence for not performing a ritual correctly or to its completion. When it comes to publishing a magazine, no ritual is involved in protecting someone from tragedy except to ensure everything in the magazine is correct so no one will experience a tragedy. Should a reference point be incorrect, a life could be lost because they may find themselves at the wrong place at the wrong time. Even worse, if there is a speck on an ad where there is not supposed to be a speck, I might not get paid for the placement.

Early in the business while living in New Orleans, I spent hours on an ad trying to determine if there was a random dot floating in the ad. It was not on any line, just in the space of the background. I brought out a magnifying glass, a photography loupe, asked my wife, and debated myself into a struggle on the front porch of my home. Without having any changes made, I took the magazine proofs to the downtown post office to send off to the printer. I made it halfway there, and, with the Superdome in sight, I started thinking I should indeed have it corrected.

"Have what corrected?" I asked myself.

"The dot, damn it, the dot."

"What dot? There is no dot."

"The hell there isn't, I saw it." I turned the car around and headed back west on I-10. While heading home I desperately asked myself, "What on earth am I doing?" I decide to turn back around and head downtown again. The Superdome was coming into view over the next overpass but I decided once again to go home and fix the damn dot.

Once home, I looked at my wife and told her I just spent the last 45 minutes driving up and down the interstate debating on whether or not to send the proofs to the printer. I told her I had decided to ask my designer to fix the dot, and she asked, "What dot?"

Then, just after the temptation to explode subsided, I realized what was so unimportant and forgetful by everyone else held the weight of the world in worry for me.

Years later, I was sitting in my psychiatrist's office pointing to a huge problem on my magazine's map. "See here," I said, "where there is no green, but just blue," (the green indicated land and the blue indicated water) "if a boat is in danger at sea and thinks this is a pass into a coastal lake, they might venture in there for safety. When they find there is no pass into the small lake, it may be too late to turn back and they could perish."

My doctor gave me a look making me realize that no boat in danger in the Gulf of Mexico would reference a tourist guide for safe havens. Nevertheless, I had it fixed, but it did not make me sleep any better because another obsession had surely taken its place.

Sex

All of my life, I dreamed of marrying a beautiful woman and having an incredible sexual relationship with her. At about the time of puberty (I hate that word), however, OCD began its stranglehold on my life. I would think about being in bed with my beautiful wife and about to do some incredible move, when all of a sudden I would have to perform a ritual and ruin the moment. As I grew older and began dating, I found this was the least of my worries. Finding a woman that would actually marry me, or at least go out with me more than three times was the more immediate challenge.

OCD crept into every moment of courtship, whether it was picking a lady up or dropping them off. I was usually late picking up my dates because my car had to be cleaned, inside and out. Not that my date would care what my car looked like (I was good looking enough), but it had to be done. On those dates I would do uncalled-for things because they had to be done, like open an umbrella when it wasn't raining, saying something completely inappropriate, trying to steal kisses at inopportune times and taking some things way too personally.

Then there were dangerous rituals: insisting my eyes were closed during make out sessions while driving, kissing with my eyes open during times of passion, or having sex without a condom – Ha! I never did that. I never had sex with anyone until marriage, but I did have my chances. If I did have sex with someone, I would have most certainly gotten her pregnant, and probably with twins. A condom would never have worked! It would have had a hole in it for sure, and I would have suffered greatly from performing endless rituals to ensure this person was not with child.

There were times I could have taken it to the limit with some ladies, but OCD made me procrastinate to the point where one fell asleep, another sobered up, and another told me to get the hell out and not come back until I grew up! (That one hurt the most.)

On one such occasion, a lady came over to my apartment on a Saturday night after I had come home without any luck with the other ladies. But there she was at my door, and then suddenly on top of me on the couch. I pretended like I was too drunk to unzip her dress, so she just got up and left. I wanted to stop her and point at my crotch and say, "Well, then, what am I supposed to do with this?" But I did not, because of being afraid of what she might say, good or bad. The worries, however, did not stop because of never going all the way. Any intimacy could be laden with bad consequences.

While at the University of Florida for graduate school, I

had given blood at the Blood Mobile on its visit to campus. After the procedure was done, they gave me a number to call if for any reason I felt my blood was tainted. Can you imagine anyone giving blood knowing it is bad?

I carried that number around with me for the maximum time required. I think it was five days. I obsessed endlessly of having AIDS. I even went as far as almost stopping by the blood center to tell them so. The fear was so daunting it kept me from thinking of anything else. I tossed and turned in bed, and could not study or socialize with friends knowing my blood would eventually kill someone.

The great thing about this obsession was that it did have a deadline, and the obsession passed along with it. However, the obsession of me having AIDS was not gone for good, and came up again as the days ticked away before my wedding.

I was living in Singapore at the time, and my wife-to-be was still in the United States. The wedding was only a few weeks away, and I felt I should call her to let her know I was at-risk. In truth, there was no way I could be at-risk, but I thought about other women I had been with and the things we did might have possibly led to me getting the disease. The chances were one in one hundred trillion, but I could never know. I sat out on the back porch of my house and argued with myself for hours. "You have it. You don't."

"You should be checked. No, you shouldn't."

"You should call your fiancé and tell her."

"Oh, no you won't."

The argument was agonizing and painful, but the real

embarrassment was mentioning it to my fiancé about a week before the wedding. She looked at me like I was crazy and let it slip by without comment. I mentioned it to her because I needed her to become involved in my obsession. She did not take the bait, and thank you God for that.

Involving someone else in an obsession makes completing rituals extremely difficult, especially because of they no know nothing of their participation. My wife has come closest to anyone who has become involved. When we used to take walks on the golf course surrounding our home, we would stick to the cart paths. You would think this would be pretty harmless, but there are expansion cracks in the path.

With OCD, "step on a crack, break your mother's back" is no longer a game; it is assumed reality. During most of our three-mile walk, I tried to time her steps with mine and ensure we stepped over a crack at the same time. If she happened to step onto a crack, I would have to start the ritual over. Even if she did step over the crack, I could not be sure if I did not step on it, because, after all, I could not be watching her foot and mine at the same time. The game went on and on for the duration of the exercise.

It is a shame, because even though she spoke the entire time, I never really listened because I was busy playing games. Although, do husbands really listen to their wives when they babble on and on during a walk? Spy any couple walking down the street, and see who is talking, and who is looking down or ahead. Most always, it is the person with the matching outfit doing all the talking.

My wife did become involved with one of my most stressful obsessions because I talked to her about it. She had no idea how much the situation had overtaken my thoughts, but I believe it almost drove me to the brink of insanity. She also did not know about my OCD, so she actually took it seriously and made me realize how stupid it was of me to even consider performing a ritual to prevent the consequence.

9/11

When obsessions involve people and the ritual performed affects them and me, someone turns out the fool, and it was always me. This particular obsession involved 9/11. That murderous day brought so much stress to this country, and so much stress on individuals. One of the triggers of my obsessions was stress, and that day there was plenty.

Although my wife and I managed to go to New York the Christmas after the mass murder, my mental state was quite stabilized. I think at the time I realized the pain inflicted on the country was so real, my obsessions, for the time being, were muted by the extreme reality.

I toured the city with blinders and tried not to look at the bulletin boards full of pictures of missing persons, although I did bring myself to look at some of them. We even visited Ground Zero, and there I also abstained from obsessing. The grief was too great to be focused on myself. I remember seeing coroner vehicles waiting to pick up any human remains that were found, and we visited a church where I gave money.

Temporary escape from my obsessions was a relief, but the reason for it was devastating.

Back at home the news was all about the failure of our government agencies to connect the dots of illegal activity. Where did we go wrong in not detecting the terrorists while they were training, and why had we not deported them when we saw their travel visas had expired? Everyone tried in vain to go about their business, but no one could have been 100% committed with the thoughts of the 9/11 terrorist attacks weighing heavily on their minds.

One day, I was making a sales call, and we were all talking about the attacks and the details of the terrorists getting access to our country's inner workings. During the conversation, the customer mentioned one of his workers had showed him an allegedly fake passport he had purchased somewhere in Central America and that this passport helped him get a job. My heart sank, my blood pressure dropped, and I surely grew faint. The gentleman who was with me let it go with a shrug and the conversation moved on to something else.

I had the weight of the world on my shoulders. I knew a person who knew a person who knew of a place in Central America churning out fake passports. If I could let the authorities know, my country would not suffer another attack. I obsessed over this for months, and the ritual would have been to talk to the employee's boss, then he would talk to the employee, the employee would reveal his sources and Green Berets would descend on the sweatshop-fake-passport factory in Central America. The weight would then be off my shoulders, and I could rest in peace. That is one of the many problems of OCD – it is all about me!

The reality of the ritual probably would have gone like this: I would have told the guy's boss, the boss would have tossed me out of his office, and someone would have for sure lost their job. That someone would have most certainly been me, and it would not have been just my job but my entire business.

It was a good thing I spoke with my wife, because she basically told me what I already knew. She told me I was nuts to even think that way. The trouble was, however, whether it was about a future terrorist attack or my mother breaking her back, I was nuts anyway. I needed someone to weed me out of this obsession. I could overcome most obsessions with stupid rituals, but since this one had something seemingly real attached to it, it took another person to relieve me of it by telling me if I acted on my decided ritual involving real people, only bad could come of it.

In the end, only bad came out of every ritual, and that was a lot of wasted time. I hate to think of the time I spent in my life obsessing over things that would have never resulted in negative consequences.

At Least Three Cookies

One of my favorite things about being an adult is I can eat cookies whenever I like. Sometimes, before I can even get used to the kitchen lights on a day of waking up before dawn, I have a cookie in my mouth. As I cook dinner, and head to the pantry, the cookie package comes into view with the enhanced picture of a chocolate chip cookie in the foreground of a fountain of chocolate cascading from a chef's wooden spoon. The temptation is too great, and I grab at least three cookies and chomp them down,

At *least* three cookies? That means to reach the "at least," the cookies must be completely whole with not a crumb missing. If there were a crumb missing, or even a molecule of a crumb missing, then there would not have been at least three cookies. There would have been 2.999999999 cookies. Deciding that I had not eaten at least three on the first attempt, four had to then be consumed; because at least three is anything greater than three. In conclusion, seven cookies usually had to be eaten before I met the "at least three" requirement. So for me to eat at least three cookies, seven had to be consumed.

The act of eating at least three was especially hard when it came to eating potato chips from the bottom half of the bag. Chips at that point are at best in halves, but mostly in quarters and eighths, and they are hard to measure considering potato chips are not measured universally (except Pringles). I would have to carefully examine chips, or pieces thereof, a number of times, and individually, to ensure I would have at least three. Since the first attempt, like that of the cookies, is never successful, I would guess a handful would be at least three. If a crumb got away or a piece of a chip escaped from my fist and onto the floor, I would have to get another fistful just to make sure I met the "at least three" requirement.

If I were eating M&M's or peanuts, I would usually have to fist at least 10, which meant on the second attempt, there would have to be 11. Since that was a high number, and counting could not be depended upon to always be correct, I would have to go to 11 one more time to ensure at least 10 were consumed. So to consume 10, I had to eat at least 32.

Would you believe I'm 5' 10" and only weigh 160 lbs.?

Playing Tennis

Tennis offers almost as many opportunities to perform rituals as does driving. There are lines to step over or on, balls to bounce and toss, a net to tap, windscreens to rub, rackets to slam on the ground and gates to open and close.

Tennis takes lots of concentration and discipline. Half the game is in your head, and that was my biggest weakness. OCD directly affected my partners or opponents because they had to wait on me to complete a ritual before beginning play.

I was an avid tennis player growing up and still play regularly. Amazingly enough, I won the 1983 Class-A Georgia state single's championship, even with a bunch of crap running through my head. I was not good because it came naturally, but because other people were dedicated to my success and happy to help me improve. One such person was a former place kicker for the Auburn Tigers in the 1950's. He was a very good tennis player and happy to play against a 16-year old.

During one of our matches, I had to stand against the fence and shoot 100 birds at myself before continuing play. He asked if I had a blister, and I said no and was embarrassed. I thought counting to 100 would be possible without him noticing the wait. I feel guilty to this day wasting that man's precious time. I wonder how many other people would like to have their time back that I wasted. I would like my time back, and I bet his family had wished he had had that little sliver of extra time to spend with them. He died of a heart attack just a few years later, and I took precious time of his life to perform a useless ritual.

In other matches, prior to serving, I would sometimes have to bounce the ball a certain number of times, hit a spot on the court with my ball bounce or draw an imaginary question mark symbol with my right foot. Just to prove how stupid all of this stuff was, I would never perform a ritual during play when the outcome of a ball placement really mattered because that is when a consequence would truly affect the outcome – winning or losing a point.

A significant problem with tennis is you can't play it alone. If I couldn't find an opponent, I would go hit balls against a wall. The practice wall at the public courts in Lagrange, Georgia was actually a handball court with a solid concrete block wall with terraced walls down each side. Hitting the ball really hard was a lot of fun, because it never really went out, and even when hitting below the line symbolizing the net, the ball always came back. The ball always coming back presented a problem though, because I was not able to leave the court until I won the last point. In reality, there is no way to win the last point against a wall, but OCD does not accept reality. Somehow, I would come up with scenarios of how I could win a point against the wall. I would hit the ball down the line, or try putting away a cross-court topspin backhand. The most common winner was to hit the ball high on the wall, and then hit an overhead. The frustrating thing about that was sometimes I would hit the ball too high on the wall, and it would go over. I would either have to wait for the person on the other side to hit it back or retrieve it myself. Even after positively winning the point, my mind would go into the evil reconciliation of convincing myself that if the "winning" shot was actually against a real opponent on a real tennis court, it would have been returned. Therefore, my 30-minute practice session would turn into a miserable hour of trying to win a point impossible of winning. When I finally did "win" the point, valuable time was spent convincing myself that there was no way an opponent could return that shot. On the walk back to my car, I passed six tennis courts, so it was a long debate.

In one situation, OCD may have helped my game. When practicing my serve with a bucket of balls, I could not quit until placing at least 10 balls in the service court (actually eleven balls – similar to the cookie count). Debates came up if one of my serves hit the net cord, and I would usually lose that debate and have to start all over again. The worst was when I missed on the 11th – the one that made it at least 10, and then have to start over. With the anxiety build-up as the number neared 10 in-a-row, the situation would almost mimic an actual pressure situation in a real match, and this probably helped me in tight matches where my serve was critical to winning, or to keep from losing.

I did the same thing in practicing basketball free shots, where I had to hit 10 in a row. I don't think I ever made 10 in a row. However, other rituals were performed: a "fuck you once" or "fuck you twice" or shooting birds at myself would have prevented any world tragedies, so the world has me to thank for either making 10 in-a-row or solving the problem in another way. "You're welcome."

One day I was shooting baskets with a little seven-year old girl. Even with a lowered rim, she could barely get the ball through the hoop. Like any child, she had a short attention span and suddenly quit playing basketball and went on to something else. I admired her greatly, because she walked away from the game after missing her last shot. I only wish I had the willpower she had.

As a person with OCD, I am able to spot other people with it. Commentators refer to those people as superstitious, but I believe it probably is OCD because the routine is the same. Many baseball players stutter step over lines on their way to the mound or back to the dugout, and many tennis players do the same when they head to mid-court between games or beyond the baseline to serve or receive. They obsess over the line, and step over it as a ritual to prevent a consequence. Is it superstition or OCD? What is the difference in this instance? They are concentrating on something other than the desired end result, which is winning.

The Movies

For many years, I did not attend movies for a number of reasons. First, the multiplex theaters were invented turning large viewing areas into small ones. The more movies showing in one location only meant fewer seats, smaller screens and terrible sound systems. I also grew bored in most movies, but the main reason, I am sure, was my OCD.

Movies were extremely exhausting experiences, because, like TV, the picture moves and changes constantly. I had no control over the speed of scenery or angle changes, so rituals would have to be performed on top of rituals to keep up with the obsessions. The first parts of the movies were particularly demanding. I know more about the opening credits than most anyone, because, while most viewers were watching the action of the opening scene, I would be having to read all of the words on the screen: Starring: ...., Produced by: ...., Executive Producer: ...., Movie Title:............, Casting Director:............, Screenplay written by: ...., Musical

Score by: ...., Costumes designed by: ....,
Based on the Story by:.........., Director of Photography:
............., Edited by: ...., Directed by:........., and they
could keep going, too. In some movies they can last for many
minutes, giving me plenty of chances to make up for earlier
mistakes, or they would end quickly causing me to wait for the
closing credits to complete a ritual.

After the credits were over, I would begin to play games
with the scenes, camera directions and characters. I would have
to do a certain number of things while looking at the eyes of the
characters, and things mattered such as a straight-on shot or a
profile shot. A character would sometimes have to be in the
frame by themselves or with other people. Sometimes I could
perform a ritual while the camera switched back and fourth
between characters, but I could not complete a ritual if the
movie went to another scene. If a ritual was not complete when
a scene changed, I could finish as long as I completed another
ritual in the next scene. This sometimes carried forward into a
number of scenes, and I would lose count as to where I was in
completing rituals for past scenes. This activity would become
quite tiresome and the anxiety would become extremely
overwhelming.

Movies are not like the tennis court, sidewalk or road. I
could not turn back to the place I was before to complete a
ritual, because the film kept moving. Thank goodness, then, for
VCRs, DVRs and DVD players. With the remote controls for
those machines, I could control the picture with the fast-
forward and rewind buttons making a 90-minute movie last for

three or more hours. Whenever my wife would watch a movie with me, I would make sure she had possession of the remote controls. It is quite unusual for a man to give the TV remote to his wife, but she never suspected why.

Reading

Reading was never one of my strong points growing up. I always enjoyed browsing through newspapers and magazines but did not like books. I blame a lot of it on my teachers picking out really boring books – the "Classics" as they called them. Any book with accompanying Cliffs' Notes was clearly not worth reading. My sixth-grade teacher had a pretty good book list. I can still remember, however, ending most of my oral book reports with, "… and if you want to find out the ending, you have to read it yourself." The belief in my teachers thinking I had read a book to the end was pretty weak, but I would give it a shot anyway.

Once my OCD struck at age 14, reading was completely out of the question. Even if I wanted to read, my brain would almost always try to keep me from enjoying a novel or article. I suffered through a number of books during my 20's and 30's only because they were page-turners: *Wild Swans*, *Into Thin Air* and *Misery*. As I got older, and the OCD got worse, the most common ritual was to finish a page or paragraph without blinking my eyes. The longer the paragraph was, the more likely for me to abuse myself. I would struggle to keep my eyes open for as long as possible before they would absolutely dry out. I was afraid for the health of my eyes and would vision an optometrist during a future eye exam telling me I had 80-year old eyes in a 50-year old body. No matter though, because the obsessions were too great and the consequences too harsh for me to worry about my own eyesight.

While living in New Orleans, my wife took me to a Barnes and Noble bookstore. After tearing myself away from the comic-strip books and the sex-help isles, I found myself in the history section. For some reason, I pulled a book called, *The Rise and Fall of the British Empire*. In some respects, this book probably played a part in saving my life. It was the thickest book I ever wanted to read and with very few pictures. Which brings up a point of something that really annoys me: These enormous books have sections of pictures in them, and they do not even count as page numbers. Once going through the picture section, the following page only increases by one page number from the page preceding the picture section. What a rip off! I think a cheap progression of page numbers is due after already reading 500 pages.

Since the book was the thickest I ever wanted to read, I never would have finished it had it not been for me seeking out a cure to OCD. When first beginning this historical behemoth, I would usually only make it through one page before having to put it down. The language in it was sometimes difficult to understand, and I could never get through a page without blinking, or stopping to ask my wife at least three times the meaning of a certain word. The book was way over my head, but I was determined to finish it.

The length of the book did, however, bring me to the realization that I would never be an avid reader with OCD. While reading a paragraph, I could see the end of the paragraph within the scope of my vision, and I would fight the natural reflex to blink when my eyes began to dry. Dryness set in first, then the stinging, and the muscles holding my eyes open would begin to give way to the reflex. Having one or two lines to go, my first strategy would be to squint my eyes to try to add moisture. When that didn't work, and it never did, I would then open my eyes wide to give me more time to finish the paragraph before the blink. Beating the reflex was almost impossible, but sometimes I was successful. It is always hard to complete a ritual when the very brain demanding I do so also insists I obey a natural reflex. It's just not fair!

There is almost nothing worse than to nearly make it all the way through a difficult paragraph and then have to start over because I blinked before reading the last word. When I returned to the beginning of the paragraph, another strategy came into play: I would begin the paragraph squinting my eyes so as not to completely expose the cornea to dry air. I never had any scientific evidence this would have a positive result, but it seemed like a good idea. Another strategy, I just thought of as of this writing, would be to sit next to a stream of vapor released from a water vaporizer. I wonder if any scientific experiments like this have been done for idiots with OCD looking for ways to fight the reflex of blinking eyes when becoming dry.

Sometimes accomplishing the feat of reading an entire paragraph without blinking was still not enough. To prevent doubt of reading the last word without blinking, I would have to read the first line of the next paragraph before blinking. Sometimes, it would have to be the first sentence of the next paragraph, and, if not successful, I could not be sure of reading the entire previous paragraph without blinking and would have to start all over again. And I thought I could read the entire history of the British Empire with OCD. After five years, and after beginning medication for my OCD, I finally finished the book.

Environments affect book reading as well. The problem with OCD is that nothing ever gets by me, and I notice everything. I would be the perfect witness to a crime if I had been present at the time of the act. Everything is noticed, because in the games of OCD, everything comes into play. Any room would do to provide obstacles to prevent the enjoyment of a book or magazine. A good example would be a waiting room at a doctor's office. Believe it or not, there is a lot of action taking place where there a bunch of people just sitting around looking bored as hell.

First, I would establish that something is happening before it would become part of the game and include that activity as an opponent in the race to finish a paragraph. If the activity occurred before I finished a paragraph in a book, I would have to start over. When my ears would detect noises, I would have to finish reading a paragraph before I would hear the following:

1. The entrance door opening,
2. The entrance door latching,
3. The nurse calling someone to, "Come on back,"
4. Someone getting paged over the loudspeaker,
5. A child sneezing, again,
6. A red neck using bad grammar, again,
7. The nurse behind the counter saying, "Fill out this form,"
8. The lady in front of me coughing,
9. The fish-tank filter making a gurgling noise, again,
10. The door from where the nurse makes the call clicking shut, or was that the front door latching? The game only gets more intriguing when the debates begin.

The doctor's office also has visible objects to distract from reading and rereading paragraphs. For example, I would finish a paragraph and then trying to prove or disprove what I saw, or didn't see, out of my peripheral vision. The object could be anything, including the following:

1. A crack in the grout in the tile floor,
2. A crack in the tile,
3. A crack in the wall,
4. A rip in the pleather couch beside me,
5. A person turning the page of a magazine,
6. Someone walking in front of me,

7. Someone's shoe on a crack in the tile,
8. A chair leg on the grout in the tile floor,
9. A crack in the ceiling tile,
10. A car passing by. Or was it a truck? Another debate begins.

Another painful aspect of reading was the necessity of having to read every single word, whether it was important or not. Good examples are footnotes and listings of names and minute details. If there were a footnote on the page, I would have to read it, no matter what. That is too bad, because I should have taken advantage of the fact that footnotes take up space on a page and make the page shorter to read. Speed-readers are able to skip unimportant details and get the point of a story and quickly move on, but reading every word to me was mandatory, even though it was pointless. Knowing it was pointless and a waste of time, I would become very anxious.

The last paragraph of a book is always the most difficult for me, and sometimes it needs to be read two or three times before closing the book for the last time. The anxiety of actually coming to the end of a book makes me not want to finish it without having to perform the ritual of reading the last paragraph a number of times.

Thank goodness I started on a drug regiment before beginning to read more history books, or having to read the bibliographies and the indexes would have been mandatory.

Reading every word of a book affected me greatly in college. Before an exam, I would force myself to read entire chapters for which the test would cover. Professors, 99% of the time, test to their lectures and not the textbooks. At Auburn University, I remember looking out the window of my room on a Saturday at my friends having fun at the Kappa Alpha Mansion. Fun I could have joined, too, but I insisted on reading the chapters. By test time, I would have read all the chapters, but still would barely pass the test.

Museums

I really hated going to museums because I would never actually get to see the exhibit. Most of my time in a museum would be spent reading the didactic placards (the signs introducing entire exhibits or sections thereof) and the labels (the little signs explaining an individual display). For example, when going through a museum in London, I came upon the Rosetta Stone. I had tirelessly read and studied about it in grade school, and pretty much had a good idea of what it was. Seeing it in real life should have been quite exciting except that the label was a full few pages long, and I spent most of my time reading it instead of looking at the rock.

Even at a museum where I had no interest in an exhibit, I had to stop and read all of the placards and labels. If I were with a group in a maritime museum, I would be left behind reading about a nail or plank of wood when they would already be looking at the reconstruction of some famous ship.

The same rules applied as in reading a book: I would have to read without blinking, and read every word.

Reading each label is very tedious because they possibly include all of the following: approximate age of the object, explanation of the object, its scientific name, from what human era or geological era did it come, from what museum it is on loan and its address, from whom it was donated by and when, and where or when was it discovered and by whom was it discovered. After having to read all of this information, who has time to actually observe the object on display?

Of all the museums I have had the pleasure of visiting while having OCD, including the Louvre in Paris, Museum of Natural History in Chicago, Museum of Ancient History and the Imperial War Museum in London, the Smithsonian in Washington, DC and the D-Day Museum in New Orleans, I, unfortunately, rarely looked at the incredible exhibits themselves but only the labels. The worst part about it was trying to make someone believe I was actually interested in an exhibit as I read its placard over and over again.

If, at a later time in the museum, I obsessed over a certain exhibit, I would have to backtrack to reread the placards. Should that have been impossible because of the flow of the crowd or having to be readmitted, other rituals like reading another exhibit's placards three or four times without blinking would have to be performed.

About five years into my treatment, I toured the Vatican. Thank goodness my pills were working, because I had to get by thousands of exhibits just to get to the Sistine Chapel. My plane was leaving Rome within a couple of hours and I had to see Michelangelo's ceiling-paint job before leaving Italy. I made it, and the only exhibit I stopped to see was the "Thinker," and I did not even read the label!

The Radio

Songs bring back memories because of their association to some special or not-so-special time. With OCD, I would intentionally tie bad things to songs I liked. Whenever one of my favorite songs came on the radio, I would say to myself something like, "Every time I hear that song, I am going to think of a soldier being killed in Iraq," or "I am going to think of the time my wife was upset over something I said."

Another ritual performed when hearing a likable song on the radio was to check all the other stations to see if there was another I liked better. After scanning through the religious stations, public radio and the obscure stations at the lower end of the dial, my preferred song would have already ended.

The same obsession applied to television while watching a particular show or a video on VH1 or MTV (they used to actually air music videos). Upon seeing something that was appealing, I would have to check all the other stations (hundreds possibly) before coming back to the station where the song or program was probably already over. Oh, how I would long for the days when my TV only got three channels.

Surprisingly the radio actually played a huge part in saving my life. One random day, while listening to "The Dennis Prager Show," a discussion relevant to my mental situation materialized. Perhaps it was the hand of God that kept my hand from touching the dial to find something "better" to tune-in.

The Rerun

_____

Sometimes, I am lucky my mind drifts off and away from the silly games and rituals. During the moments of seemingly peaceful solitude, my brain actually becomes relaxed and floats off into a distant world where relaxation is reality. But then, "Oh, no! Did I just run a stop sign at that last intersection? I could have killed someone had there been another car or someone crossing the street. Whew, I guess I made it. Everything seems to be ok. I really should be more careful, but I wonder if I really could have hurt someone. Oh well, it does not really matter, nothing is wrong." Anxiety suddenly builds inside of me, and I turn the car around.

I will go back to check out the situation *not* to see if I did kill anyone, but to see if it was possible I could kill someone and to make sure even the possibility did not exist. This is one of the more odd obsessions, because there was no evidence of an accident (no screeching of tires). Just to think the possibility an accident could occur in the future if I were to run the stop sign at that intersection is enough to make me have to go back.

Arriving back at the intersection, I discover there is no stop sign, so everything is cool. At the next intersection, I run a yellow light. I obsess again that I could have, but only possibly, caused an accident. In this situation, I have to turn the car around and drive through the light again, but this time when it is green. By doing this rerun, I conclude that having an accident at this intersection is possible, but running a yellow light would not be the cause.

Reruns sometimes involve other people's lives as well. When a bunch of friends did some tubing behind my boat, I was worried of pulling one of the riders too close to the pilings of a dock. After the initial pass, I pictured what *could* have happened: As the rider bounced over the boat's wake and made the slingshot to the other side toward the dock, she would have had no control over the speed and direction as the pilings fell right into her path. With the rope tight and the motor at full throttle, she would have slammed into the wooden pilings and broken her neck and been sliced up by barnacles. Just to make sure this could not have happened on the first run, I took another pass at a similar distance to ensure myself the distance was appropriate and an accident like that could not possibly happen.

Downhill snow skiing is one of the most wonderful sports invented. It could be the most perfect sport, because everything is literally downhill all the way, and the ski lifts do the real work in taking you uphill. One of my favorite mountains to ski is Copper Mountain in Summit County,

Colorado. To begin my first day of skiing, I would wake up in LaGrange, Georgia at 4:30 a.m., dress in my ski clothes, and be on the plane in Atlanta by 7 a.m. By 11:30 a.m., I would be in the lift line at the ski resort. Four whole days of skiing, and, after the first few hours, I think to myself, "Gosh, I wish this trip would hurry up and end."

Skiing alone, while suffering with OCD, is not relaxing because of the freedom I have to choose my own routes and speeds. There is no one to follow and no one to lead – just the wide-open expanse of OCD all to myself. "Where's that jump?" is a phrase heard by some on the slope, and I found a jump that was fairly satisfying near the end of a blue run. "Here it comes! Traverse, traverse, tuck, hit it, spread eagle and land. That was good, but not perfect. I need to tuck sooner."

Back in the lift line I go, on the chair, off the chair, down the first part of the hill, cut hard to the second part, and now down the final slope, "Traverse, traverse, tuck, hit it, spread eagle and land. Damn it, too slow again. Maybe I need to spring off the jump harder."

Back to the lift, down the run to the final slope, "Tuck, hit it, spread eagle, land. Perfect. Now let's go try some other runs, maybe hit some black mogul runs. No, lets do that jump again and really feel myself getting airborne."

"Cut, traverse, traverse, tuck, hit it, look left and right, land. Still not good, so do it again." This would go on for hours until I would either have enough courage to end the repetition, or the ski lift would eventually close on schedule at 4:00 p.m. Oh, well, I still have three more days to "enjoy" myself.

Waterslides are fun, too, except for having to walk up to the top without having the aid of a chairlift.

"Ok, here we go and I really need to get the out-of-body experience and feel myself going down the flume and coasting up and down the edges before I hit the pool at the bottom."

Back up to the top, and, "Ok, again, but this time, really try to feel the excitement and speed."

Climb the stairs again, and, "This time down, notice the sides flying past you and really feel the rush."

Another climb to the top, and, "This time down, really concentrate on the water you are gliding on and that you are actually speeding down with it." I think to myself, "How long before this waterpark closes?"

Thank you God that Lewis and Clark never had to complete reruns because of silly obsessions, or they never would have made it even to the Midwest. I guess the only good place to have this kind of problem is on the roller rink or a racetrack. Maybe that is the reason NASCAR drivers seem so happy doing what they do.

The Follow-up

When being taught strategies to become successful in life, people say you should always follow-up. In basketball, you should follow your shot in case you miss; in tennis, you should follow your approach shot to the net; in courting, you should follow-up the night after a date to make sure she had fun; after receiving free tickets from a friend, you should follow-up to let them know you really appreciated the great seats; when job hunting, you should follow-up with the employer after the interview to let them know you are interested; in sales, you should follow-up with the potential customer to make sure they are interested.

In my world of OCD, I always follow a derogatory comment or a regretful story with a positive or somber note. This falls in the same category as not walking off the basketball court until making the last shot, or ensuring the last joke told is received well by listeners. Departing impressions are almost as important as first impressions. (I always feel sorry for retiring or graduating quarterbacks, who, on the last throw of their career, throw an interception.)

While living in Australia, I visited the Outback in my company car. It was a station wagon I used for carrying carpet samples and was not at all built for driving around in the desert. After having the radiator rebuilt on the way out there and my water hoses replaced on the way back, I met face to face with a kangaroo with only the windshield between us. Since I was going pretty fast at the time, my car was badly damaged and the kangaroo died. I felt awful.

Shortly after the accident, two locals appeared and noticed I was quite upset. They rushed over to me and said they would check things out. They went straight to my car, lifted the bonnet (hood) and examined the engine. "No worries, mate. Engine looks good. You'll be right to go."

I there stunned while looking at them. I said, "What about the kangaroo?" They looked back at me kind of puzzled, walked over to it and said, "He's dead, mate." My concern was with the animal; they were concerned about the car. Fact is, there were dead kangaroos all up and down the highway, and Australian transport trucks are built with "Roo Bars" to knock them off the road without doing harm to their vehicles. My little station wagon only had a plastic bumper. I had killed a kangaroo; I felt terrible, and my boss was going to kill me.

Of course, word got out around Sydney about what had happened. It was hard to hide the wounds of my automobile. Friends started calling me "Roo Russell." They would tell others why they called me that, and I would have to tell the story. The tale got back to the States through the grapevine of my company and filtered to my family and friends. It made for a good story, people always wanted to hear of it, and I enjoyed telling of my great experience in the Outback. However, I always had to end the story with, "But I sure felt bad about that kangaroo." Truth is, I did feel bad for that kangaroo, but having to throw that phrase in at all costs was only an obsession. I would be in the middle of the story and throw it in at inappropriate times. Otherwise, if I had told the story without revealing my feelings of killing an innocent animal, I would mention it later in the conversation or even later in the night. People would look at me and sometimes wander what the hell I was talking about.

Moreover, it had to be said to everyone within earshot of the story. I would obsess about it at a particular gathering until I was sure everyone knew my feelings about killing that animal. My evenings at a large dinner table would be ruined, and I would even look like a bigger idiot when getting out of my chair to go to someone at the other end of the table to make sure they heard me say, "But I sure felt bad about that kangaroo."

Other examples of the follow-up include things said about people – especially dead ones. Growing up and being an Auburn fan, I can always say something derogatory about Bear Bryant. Every time I did, though, I would follow it up with, "But he was a great coach."

The following list shows where the first part of the phrase is the opinion and the second part is the act of the obsession-satisfying follow-up ritual:

1. That guy sure is such an ass, but he means well.
2. She sure is ugly but very nice.
3. He is a terrible tennis player but he tries.
4. He is loosing his hair but he still gets the ladies.
5. She is a real snob but good at what she does.
6. He sure is a dick, but he has a nice car. (Not really a good example, but I heard it said about someone I know and thought it was pretty funny!)
7. Captain Morgan was a truly evil man, but he was a successful buccaneer.
8. My boss is a jerk to work for, but his heart is in the right place.
9. His wife is so selfish, but she does a good job raising the children.
10. She is a serial killer. Bless her heart.

The act of completing a ritual by saying the second part of the phrase is meant to release me of any guilt or of the consequence of hurting someone's feelings, even though that someone is either far from the conversation, dead or actually a truly horrible person.

Relaxation

Relaxation has no place in the life of someone with OCD. OCD'rs must always be busy. Even when it looks like we are relaxed, we are hard at work.

When my psychiatrist asked me what successfully controlling my OCD looked like, I told him about a man I saw on the golf course sitting in his golf cart, leg up on the dash and smoking a cigar while he waited his turn. I said, "I want to be that man." And I don't even smoke cigars, play golf or have a desire to wear mismatched clothes with white shoes and a white belt, but the guy just looked so relaxed and carefree.

Flying Kites

One of the most wonderful ways in the world to relax is flying a kite. Let the wind catch the fabric, spin the string off the spindle and away it goes into the beautiful blue sky. Gazing at its beauty while white puffy clouds float in the background is pure relaxation. Then someone had to go and invent stunt kites.

I was a stunt kite flyer long before it became a hip sport.

I was living in Sydney, Australia at the time, and the wind was always perfect there with plenty of room to fly. My friends and I would go to the kite store on Manly Beach, buy one for $100 and then spend half that much on string. We would find a secluded road and roller skate behind the kite, or a field and slide along the grass as it pulled us along under its great acceleration.

Those things were so noisy and fast; we could clear an entire section of sunbathers off a beach. If one kite was not enough, we would stack kites one above another for more speed, lift and noise. It was great fun, unless I was alone.

The simplest of stunt kites has two strings for each hand to guide the kite in different directions. By pulling on the strings, the kite can land and take off, dip its wing in the water, cut horizontally over the ground, fly straight up or straight down, or spin in tight or loose circles. The minute my kite went up in the air, my brain took over barking out orders and directions for the kite to fly. There was never any happy-go-lucky for the kite, and I would have to spin in it one direction for a certain number of times, and then unwind it to separate the strings and continue to spin it in the other direction. The kite would have to touch the ground and stay for a certain number of seconds, and I would have to do it over and over again until it met my brain's commands.

Should there have been people on the beach, I would dare to fly close to them to see if they would be disturbed. With ocean waters next to me, I would have to dip the wing in the water and bring it out, again. The colder the water, the deeper I would force myself to dip the wing, therefore bringing closer the possibility of me having to swim out to retrieve it had it not been able to lift out with the pull of the string. The sooner I met all the demands the better. Then I could go home and take a break from this "relaxing" activity.

Sailing

Sailing is absolutely one of my most favorite things to do. Since I live in Florida, the season lasts long and the opportunity to sail and teach other people to sail is a very rewarding experience. As with kite flying, it is something that should not be done alone if suffering with OCD.

I have access to three boats: a 17.5-foot Hobie catamaran, a Sunfish and a 22-foot Catalina. Each serves its purpose for the kind of passenger and current weather. For a dry sail, sunset cruise or one with older passengers, the Catalina is perfect. For exceptional wind, excitement, younger passengers and warm water, the catamaran is the ticket. For calm winds, or extremely high winds and a very wet sail, the Sunfish is the choice of the day.

The catamaran has caused most of my troubles while having OCD even though it is the boat I most prefer. During a very good wind, the windward hull is sometimes able to lift completely out of the water making the ride exhilarating and an impressive site for spectators. "Flying the hull" is the typical description of the experience. There is a point of no return during the flight, and that is when I am atop the windward pontoon and looking straight down in the water. At this point, the boat is either going to turn on its side, or, with any luck, fall back with both pontoons in the water. A milestone, before the point of no return, occurs when the windward rudder comes completely out of the water. Rather than looking forward and enjoying the flight, I would force myself to watch the rudder make its exit.

Also, I would not consider myself to be in flight unless the rudder did become free of the water. I would obsess about flying the hull even on mildly windy days, and even though I got the hull out of the water it would not be satisfactory, and I would have to continue sailing to the point of no longer enjoying what I loved doing most.

The Catalina is the best "day sailing" boat around. It can also be very boring and hot depending on the wind. On an especially cold, windy day, I decided to take it for a spin in what would be the perfect example of OCD overcoming common sense. To sail this boat alone, you must be able to walk around the boat under sail, with the tiller locked and a rope connecting you to the boat. This is particularly important in strong winds and rough water. Common sense would say to stay home and watch a movie, but OCD told me to get out there and face the dangers and consequences of stupidity.

On that particular day, I decided to combine a barge lane, a toll bridge, 25 mph wind gusts and 3-foot seas as my challenge. Not only that, but in the middle of my adventure, I found myself on the bow of the boat untangling the jib. It was very exhilarating and made for a good story (I never told my father, though, because it was his boat, after all). When it was over, I obsessed for days about how I could have killed myself or rammed the boat into the bridge destroying it. All out of an obsession to face the danger, and on the next cold, windy day, I did a rerun to make sure what I did was not really a potential life killer or boat sinker. The boat and I survived, but it was no fun and a stupid thing to do.

On both the catamaran and Catalina, there are shrouds to play with, too. The shrouds are the wires holding the mast to the deck of the boat. With landmarks, clouds, the sun or other moving objects, I try to keep the shrouds on one side of them or the other. Birds, boats and other moving objects are particularly tough, and wooden shipping-lane markers make the game downright dangerous.

Using the alternating-blinking-eye method makes the game even more interesting by keeping an object on one side of the shroud with only my left eye open and then only my right. My passengers must have often wondered why I committed to going one direction and then suddenly jerking back to go another. Little did they know, I was saving the world from coming to an end.

My other boat is a Sunfish, which is probably one of the most fun and easiest boats to sail. I learned to sail on a Sunfish, and I believe if you can sail one of these small boats, you can sail almost any sized boat. The boat I own is one built in the 1970's, so it is considerably heavier than the later models to a tune of about 200%. The steering parts are all made of wood, and the sail is the original, now a faded yellow and orange design. It has been beat up quite a bit in hurricanes and its trailer is somewhere in the bottom of Little Sabine Bay in Pensacola, Florida. It is mostly kept togethcr with love and Marine Tex patching compound.

The obsession with the Sunfish was that I had to be able to see the wooden-dagger board when I heeled the boat. The risk in this was the same with the catamaran in that if I pushcd the envelope too far, the boat would flip. This was really no big deal, because this boat was easy to flip back. I could usually do it without getting wet just by letting the boat roll and then sliding my body up the side and stand on the dagger board and jump back in the boat when it righted itself.

The part that was so frustrating was the incredible loss of speed when heeling (professional Sunfish sailors actually put on considerable weight to ballast their boats so heeling is limited). The other was trying to force it to heel by leaning forward in a light wind and then leaning back quickly to catch a glimpse of the dagger board. The biggest loss with this obsession was the lack of enjoyment on what otherwise should be a fun experience, but I am sure the world is better off because completing the rituals has surely made the world a safer place.

Scuba Diving

Another wonderful way to relax is to go scuba diving. There is nothing like swimming deep beneath the water's surface without having to worry about coming up for air. All you need is about 120 lbs. worth of equipment. It amazes me to no end that diving has not become any lighter since the heyday of Jacques Cousteau. Oh, it is now computerized and mixed gasses make deeper diving possible, but it is still a pain to carry all of that stuff around. I never could get the tank in the right position either, and I always had trouble lifting my head. I have dived with the best of them in places like the Great Barrier Reef, the Gold Coast and in the south of New South Wales, Australia. I even dove a number of times in Sydney Harbor. I have done drift diving off the coast of Mexico, deep diving in the Gulf of Mexico and spring diving in south and northwest Florida. But the truth is, I never liked it. Every time I went out, I felt like I was never coming back to dry land. Even when I did 10-foot lake dives during my certification classes, I obsessed about dying and prayed to God for my safe return to the surface.

Since the equipment requires so many connections and working parts and other equipment, I was a firm believer in Murphy's Law that what can go wrong, will go wrong. I always had to check and double check connections, test breathe, and constantly check my dive table to ensure I was not going to get the bends.

When I was actually underwater, the fun really began. I would act as I did when first seeing a naked Bo Derek and kid myself this was the most wonderful experience and the most beautiful view. My tank gauge was always in my left hand and I checked it constantly: on the way down, at the bottom and on the way up. One time, I was so consumed by watching the gauge, that I was poking my dive partner in his side with my spear gun. Man, did he ever make a mean face at me.

I would force myself to spend too much time in one place examining stuff that really did not interest me. That got me in trouble in Playa del Carmen, Mexico. Since it was a drift dive, the rest of my group was moving far ahead and the guide got upset with me.

One of the most peaceful experiences, I must admit, is the safety stop 10 feet below the surface on the ascent back to the boat. I used to imagine it was a trip to heaven because the deep water was cold and the closer I got to the surface, the more pleasant it became. It was such a great feeling, and if there is any great pleasure I ever got from diving, that was it.

When my wife and I moved to Singapore and started visiting islands in the South China Sea and Thailand, we switched entirely to snorkeling!

Swinging

Swinging in swings is a wonderful pastime. You can meditate by just barely pushing your legs from the ground and gently sway back and forth. Close your eyes and feel the gentle breeze generated by the movement of your body like a pendulum in a grandfather clock relaxes the senses and frees the mind. You can also go full bore by kicking your legs and extending the chains out with your arms pushing the swing higher and higher. Sometimes you can swing so high you can pull the steel frame of the swing set from the ground and putting slack in the chain causing a jerk on the descent. This kind of swinging activity is good exercise and a nice stress reliever. But, of course, the positive results swinging may bring to someone only works for those without OCD.

One thing I look for in a swing set is its location. I would much rather find a swing set in a nice environment with a pretty view than one in a dirt lot behind a warehouse. In Sydney, Australia, there was a swing set I loved to visit at a location called McMahon's Point. It sat just west of the Harbor Bridge near North Sydney. It was also one of my favorite places to make sales calls when I did not want to go to the office. The view was much better than the sight of the dull-blue fabric of my cubicle. Other salespeople with car phones would go down there, too, and one time one of my fellow salesmen drove up behind me and called me saying, "I caught you mate."

In the evening, the view from this park could not have been more gorgeous. The emerald color of the Harbor Bridge illuminated under its powerful lights and the Sydney Opera House in view across the harbor made for a beautiful sight. Adding to the scene was the Sydney skyline in the background, and the reflection of the entire view bouncing off of the water. It was a view most people only see on a picture postcard, and others would pay dearly to experience it first hand. Not me, though. I was right there and able to enjoy it every single night, and right there in the park in a nice grassy area was a swing set offering the perfect venue from which to play the games of OCD. These games would make this incredible view one of mental torture and anxiety.

While swinging, the view changes constantly and only stays static during those milliseconds when at the top of the back end or front end of the swing before reversing the motion.

Objects in the distance can be below an object close by at the lowest part of the swing, and the same objects can be above an object close by at the highest part of the swing. Placing the objects at a certain point above or below other objects became the object of the games. Throw the crossbar of the swing set in the view at the back end of the swinging motion and another element is added to the process of my having to save the world.

After first mounting the swing and grabbing the chains, the view would be breathtaking. While swinging like a pendulum and gaining height, I would begin to obsess about having to see the top of the Opera House hidden by the bottom of the Harbor Bridge. Once accomplishing that, I would obsess about seeing the top of the Opera House above the road level of the bridge forcing me to pull and push harder on the chains resulting in my body being jolted by the slacking and tightening of the chains.

With the crossbar in play, I would attempt to have the entire Harbor Bridge appear above the structure by pushing even harder on the chains. Once accomplishing that feat, I would push harder and attempt to have the Opera House and the Harbor Bridge appear above the crossbar. The jerking would get violent, and I would wonder about the stability of the swing, but the world was dependent upon me to make the view as my brain envisioned it should be.

After accomplishing demands made upon me during the swinging, came the demands made upon me for the dismount. Knowing the dangers of jumping from a location too high, my mind would set the bar high, and I would have to see the lower parts of some of the buildings in the skyline above the bridge before jumping from the swing. If I did not see the spot demanded of me, or if I doubted I saw it, the action of swinging and jumping would have to be repeated, again and again. Of course, if it were impossible to complete a ritual, I would shoot fifty birds at myself, or something of the related sort, to ensure the safety of the world.

All this being difficult, throwing in the cars moving across the bridge and the ferryboats sliding across the water, the act of completing rituals became nearly impossible. With moving objects making time a factor in some of the games, I would have to complete the ritual before one of the boats or cars reached a certain point on the bridge or upon the water.

I always wanted to take a date down to those swings, but I never did. How much fun it could have been, and how disappointing it was to know that I would turn a beautiful experience into a miserable game.

Fast-forward twenty years, and I now have a little girl who loves to swing. I don't obsess about having her reach a certain height, or in a position where I can see certain objects behind her after ascending or descending. Since I am now on medication, there are no consequences for not completing rituals. She safely swings back and fourth, and says, "Higher, daddy, higher." I could have never imagined, when I was in Sydney, this activity could become a pleasure, but I thank God that it is for my daughter and me.

Sleeping

The ultimate form of relaxation is sleeping. It is a wonderful gift from God, but it takes up too much time. I think God made sleep necessary because it gives us less time to screw up. At least when we are asleep, He does not have to worry about us hurting ourselves or someone else.

One of the first questions my psychiatrist asked was whether or not I had a hard time going to sleep. I do not have a hard time going to sleep, but rituals had to be completed before dosing off.

Once I slipped into bed, I would try to read a book, but would usually have to stop after reading one page, or one paragraph because of the games I would play. Once I turned off my light, the most amazing peace would set in, but it would usually last only seconds. As my pupils adjusted to the darkness and my ears to the silence, I could see nothing but pitch black and hear nothing but the rustling of sheets. For a precious few seconds, there were no distractions from which to create games. Once my eyes adjusted, I could make out the outlines of the furniture and see the tree sway outside the window. My ears suddenly could hear a train in the distance and the humming of car engines from the nearby highway. All distractions reappeared.

Once my peace ended, I would say my prayers. That was also a routine, because like my showers, my prayers followed the exact-same order for 22 years. I could say that is the reason God never seemed to answer my prayers regarding OCD because He quit listening to me. I don't think He ever quit listening, but I do believe He probably listened with the dread of hearing the same rerun every night.

My prayer always ended with, "God bless America. Amen." If for some reason the end of my prayer did not agree with my current OCD game, I would have to repeat the phrase over and over again until getting it right. In that case, I do believe God did quit listening and moved on to someone else's prayers for the evening, and I hope that He did quit listening to me at that point, because I could only picture Him tapping His fingers in frustration.

If I was lucky, my night ended with sharing time with a loved one. My wife usually was in bed before I was, so I had to be very quiet slipping in beside her. After completing my prayers, my little love would come up to my side. My hand would begin to rub her from just below her neck and down her back to just above her buttocks. I would either use the palm of my hand or my fingernails. After sounds of pleasure came from deep within her, she would roll over onto her side with her back against my chest, and my hand would move in a similar manner from just below her chin, over her chest, and across her belly and then back up again. Her noises would become louder and louder, especially when she exhaled. Then, suddenly, the noises of pleasure would stop and she would get to her feet, jump off the bed and make her way to the litter box or her bowl of food. I was never sure which, because I would usually be fast asleep the second she left the room.

A Beautiful View

Traveling the world has offered me some great views: beaches on the South China Sea, Yosemite National Park, the Southern Cross, volcanoes in Indonesia and Central America, snow-covered mountains of the Rockies, New Zealand's South Island and the Alps, landmarks like the Eiffel Tower and Big Ben, the Australian Outback and topless women on beaches.

I'd like to say the first look at these things of beauty are what garnered my greatest attention towards them, but it was tearing myself away from them that brought me displeasure and pain. I had to observe them one last time, and that always involved performing rituals.

Since life does not last forever, the moment before turning away from something could be the last moment of ever seeing that something. Since the risk of never seeing something again is so great, I always wanted to make sure the last sight I had of a beautiful view was perfect.

Perfect sometimes meant making sure my feet were pointed in a certain direction, or I had to stare at the view a certain length of time without blinking. If a view was in motion, like the ocean surf, a sky full of floating clouds, or the evening air flickering with the fire of lightening bugs, I would have to make sure I looked away at just the right moment.

As my obsessions overtook my sense of wonder, beautiful views were not something I wanted to gaze at in amazement any longer, but something I just wanted to get away from. As I turned and walked away, in many cases, I would sing to myself, "Don't Look Back" by the rock group Boston. If I had known any of the other words to the song, it might have helped in keeping me from turning around.

The most painful of this kind of obsession came when visiting my grandmother in her nursing home. Her life was definitely not going to last forever, and, after every visit, I feared I would never see her again. For about ten years I thought that. She was not giving up easy and was outliving everyone else in the home. She was going through roommates like a nerd in a college dorm. The family joked that anyone moving in with my grandmother was granted their death wish, because they were bound to go before she did.

My grandmother's nursing home was in Birmingham, Alabama, and I would usually visit her on Saturdays during football season. As she grew older, the only thing she could really understand me say was Auburn University's battle cry, "War Eagle."

After stepping off the elevator, I would walk down the corridor past almost all the bedrooms on her floor. In the majority of rooms, without fail, a football game was on the occupant's television. The games were usually an Auburn or Alabama game or at least an SEC game. In the community room, residents were placed in front of the big-screen TV to watch a game. Some knew what was going on, and others just faced the screen with their eyes closed and their mouths open. One man, I remember in particular, never had his eyes open, but he always wore a crisp-clean, white Auburn hat.

When my visit was over, I would kiss my grandmother goodbye and head out the door. Convinced this was the last time I would ever see her, I would obsess all the way to her door, and then have to look at her again and possibly have to go back and kiss her again. This was a dangerous mission because one time she punched me when I went to kiss her on the cheek.

On my second attempt to leave, I would obsess and perform rituals all the way to the door. Taking a certain number of steps, looking at a family picture out of the corner of my eye, shooting birds at myself, making sure not to step on the cracks in the vinyl floor, and ensuring the correct foot exited the door first were just some of the many rituals performed.

Leaving her room and having her out of site was not the end, however. I still had to get past the nurses station, clear the community room where the man with the Auburn hat slept in front of the TV, climb the steps to the parking level (waiting on the arrival of the elevator would have only increased the time available for more obsessions and rituals), walk past the chapel and the receptionist, through the parking lot and finally arrive at my car. The obsessions ended on almost every visit on the timing of my car door closing.

From the time I left her room until I got to my car, I would have performed fifty or so rituals, so I would not have to return to her room and look at her again "one last time."

Self-Inflicted Pain

One of the biggest dangers of OCD is to injure myself to either create a greater distraction than the object of an obsession or to actually hurt myself to complete a ritual.

The latter, I believe, is the worst kind of injury because it is done after succumbing to an imaginary consequence. While living in Australia, I made an ill-advised trip in the company car to the "Red Center" from Sydney. Since Australia is only made up of six states and two territories, they have very strict rules regarding the transportation of fruit over state lines. Well, being the tightwad I am, I refused to throw my small bag of fruit in the trashcan at one of the borders. By the time I started obsessing that I alone would destroy the entire agricultural industry of South Australia with fruit from Victoria, it was too late to turn back and make things right. A few hours into South Australia, I saw a fruit fly on the inside of my window, and I worried about being deported if I got caught. I had a huge anxiety attack over that little fruit fly and almost crashed the car trying to kill it.

My obsession grew so great, I thought about calling the Agricultural Ministry. As luck would have it though, it was a holiday that day, and no one would have answered the phone. I thought about going to the police but ultimately ate what I had, threw the core and pits in a receptacle and got the hell out of that town.

On the way to Ayer's Rock, or Uluru as the Aborigines call it, I stopped in the opal capital of the world, Coober Pedy. It is a little town just inside the Northern Territory boundary where a young boy on a gold hunting expedition discovered opals. His elders sent him out to look for water, and he came back with the treasure instead.

Coober Pedy is desert country. Half of the homes and businesses there are actually underground because of the intense heat. Their golf course is made entirely of dirt and the greens are actually colored black with oil.

While walking along, I had an obsession requiring me to stare at the sun for 10 seconds without blinking. One thing about OCD is my brain usually picked the most inopportune places to perform certain rituals, especially when these rituals can cause immense and permanent damage. I performed the ritual and everything was cool. For the rest of the day, I saw spots and obsessed that my eyes were permanently damaged.

OCD does not know of the process of learning from mistakes. Almost twenty years later while my wife and I were living on a golf course in northwest Florida, a cosmos event was taking place that I wanted to witness. Living on a fairway gave me a good opportunity to view the eclipse without much obstruction. This eclipse, however, was not lunar or solar, and really not an eclipse at all, but similar to one in that Venus was crossing in front of the sun in the early-morning hours. I became obsessed with the possibility that I could actually see this tiny spec cross in front of our gigantic sun without the assistance of astronomy equipment. Using a pair of cheap sunglasses, I looked directly into the sun. For about an hour afterwards, I laid in bed with my eyes closed hoping to God the huge round-yellow ball would disappear from between my eyeball and eyelids. It was finally gone by the next morning.

The good thing about these kinds of obsessions is they can't be made right by performing a ritual, because these kinds of obsessions involve real situations, which brings me to the reason for inflicting a wound on myself: I would not have to worry about made-up obsessions but of actual physical discomfort.

Obsessions can be so painful that the only thing possibly making them irrelevant is a real problem. I often wished to contract an illness or be physically harmed so my anxiety would actually be over something real and my obsessions would become irrelevant.

At other times, I would punch my hand to the wall hoping to break a bone, or kick something with the hope of harming my foot. During the worst obsessions, physical harm to myself seemed less traumatic than having to perform rituals to prevent imaginary tragedies.

Doors

Growing up in LaGrange, Georgia in what I would consider a very nice house, I had my own room of light panel pine walls and two closets each with two hinged doors. One was for my toys and the other for my clothes and the place where I hung my Nerf basketball hoop. That hoop delayed me getting my homework started, getting dressed, going to bed, and it also woke my father countless times after he had already gone to bed. There was nothing worse than the look on my father's face when he was rudely awakened.

Long before consequences and rituals were associated with my obsessions, I insisted every night I "check my closets." At first, I would simply place my thumb between the two adjacent doors to make sure they were evenly matched. On one occasion, one of my sister's friends slept over at our house and she saw me doing it and said, "You just got to make sure, huh?"

As time moved on, I began to mash my thumb hard in between the crack to the point of having an indention in my thumb where the skin was pinched, and it was painful.

As I grew older and started staying up later than my parents, I became the door locker and checker. We had three doors to the outside that needed to be locked before going to bed. The responsibility lay with my father, so I thought, to lock the doors. I would be astonished to find sometimes they were not locked. This was his castle and he was leaving the moat bridge down!

Between the 11 o'clock news and the "Benny Hill Show," I would get up to check the locks. The door to the carport was a push button lock, and it was fairly easy to see that it was locked. I would still have to pull it to make sure it was latched and then push the button in one more time to make sure it was set. The door to the courtyard was one of those where the doorknob had to be pushed in and then turned to the right to secure the lock. The trouble with this one was not being able to see that it was locked after stepping away. I would lock it, and say to myself while looking at it, "It is locked; it is definitely locked."

The front door was a large wooden door with little windows on the side. My mother had it installed to replace the "Brady Bunch" doors. (They were hideously ugly double doors with the doorknobs in the middle of each door.) To get to the front door, I had to walk through the foyer separated from the hallway by two swinging louvered doors. They unlatched loudly from the doorframe and when opened would vibrate the entire house.

The front-door lock was a bolt lock, and was fairly easy

to see, but I had to go through the "locked, definitely locked" procedure, anyway. Upon leaving the foyer, I had to exit those doors again, and when they latched, the entire house would vibrate, again.

After the "Benny Hill Show" was over at midnight, I would repeat the door-lock process one more time. The next ritual was to check the refrigerator door to make sure it was closed. I thought that if it were not closed, all the food would spoil and drip onto the floor. I would picture my mother sitting on the floor in front of the refrigerator crying and picking up food that was now garbage, while daddy left for work and my sister and I set off to school. Therefore, making sure the refrigerator was closed was a very important ritual.

Once that process was complete, I checked the freezer in the laundry room and then went through the entire process of checking the doors one more time before going to the bathroom to get ready for bed.

One more ritual, however, had to be performed before heading to my bedroom, and that was called shaking the pipes (creating a noise with water pressure in metal pipes). After brushing my teeth, I would turn the hot water valve on and off very quickly which made a loud noise in the crawl space underneath the house. I would do this three times and swore I would quit doing it if it ever woke my father and he told me to stop. It never woke him, so I did it every night for nearly 10 years.

Once in my bedroom, I checked closets, and I went to bed with two sore thumbs.

Pool gates are also a source of high anxiety. If they are not closed correctly, a toddler would definitely die. In my business, I go through a lot of pool gates. Not because of my business with so many vacation resorts, but the fact that many easily accessible bathrooms are near pools. Being in outdoor sales and in my car most of the day, I have to steal the use of a lot of other people's plumbing for my physical comfort. Thank goodness pay toilets do not exist so much, or at all, as they once did. Like other reruns, the pool-gate obsession involves checking and rechecking the locks and then pulling excessively on the gate to ensure it can't be opened with just an easy push. Once I was convinced the gate could not be opened, I would return to my car and continue my day.

After a few minutes of driving serenity, I would suddenly picture a toddler wander through the parking lot, venture toward the pool, push the gate open, fall into the pool and drown. Family and friends of the little one would wait in desperation as first responders came to try to revive the baby but would instead pronounce the child dead. After these horrific thoughts, I would turn my car around and head back to the pool to check once again that the gate is locked. "It is locked; it is definitely locked," and another life is saved.

Dangerous Tools

A tool can be anything used to complete a mechanical, structural or construction project. Tools are also used to solve problems and accomplish certain tasks. Tools can also be very dangerous if not used correctly, and there are many ways to use a tool incorrectly.

Horror movies, "Action News at 11:00" and novels portray tools used as weapons to injure or kill another being whether a human or an animal. The most common tools shown are tire irons, hatchets, hammers, kitchen knives, screwdrivers, letter openers and scissors. In my world of OCD, all these tools are available and the victims would be my relatives, friends or my pets.

Probably the most horrible aspect of OCD is picturing the outcome of a consequence. I would actually see myself creep up to my cat, dog or mother, father, sister, wife or friend and bludgeon them with a hammer, repeatedly stab them with a screwdriver or cut them with a kitchen knife. The only time I would do this was at bedtime when I actually saw one of the tools out of place – like spotting a screwdriver on my bedside table left from an earlier project, or a hammer in the hallway where I left it when I hung pictures earlier in the day.

After spotting the misplaced tool, the vision would go through my head, and be so horrible and all too vivid. I would be sick just knowing the visions were actually in my head. I would tell myself there is no way in hell of actually following through with such a horrific act, but then I would remind myself it is certainly something that could happen were I to suddenly begin to sleepwalk. (I have never walked in my sleep.)

The ritual performed many times to prevent such carnage involved me putting the tool in a place where it would be difficult or inconvenient to reach for the purpose of wreaking havoc upon someone while walking in my sleep. If it were a screwdriver on my bed stand, I would place it in my chest of drawers underneath my underwear. If it were a hammer, I would place it at the top of my closet where it would be hard to reach. Scissors would be placed in a drawer in the bathroom. The purpose for these strange hiding places was that I would surely wake up while trying to reach them in their awkward locations.

In the most irritating situation, a writing pen could become dangerous. If I were writing in my diary in bed, I would have to throw the pen under the bed and out of reach.

Don't think I couldn't find these tools two or three weeks later when I needed them for actual work. With OCD, I never forget anything.

My belt

Living in a two-story house is ideal because the living area is truly separated from the sleeping area. Beds do not have to be made-up and bathrooms not completely clean should an unexpected guest arrive. In some older homes, most money for house upkeep is spent on the downstairs area to impress visitors while the upstairs areas are only kept in need of repair.

Stairs, however, become an obstacle when an effort is made to alleviate the possibility of choking someone to death. In my house, with a young daughter and a wife, I have been relegated to the downstairs closets for my wardrobe. I am allowed to use the clothes hamper in the master bedroom to place my just-worn outfit before changing into pajamas kept in my chest of drawers that is allowed in the master. I am, however, not allowed to place my choice of décor on top of the chest.

Anyway, should my outfit of the day include a belt, it mustn't be left upstairs where I could uncoil it and sneak up on one of my family members and choke them to death. The belt must be safely hung on its hook in my closet downstairs. I always pretend to need something from the kitchen when I take it downstairs. This action resulting in wasted time and another made-up excuse to cover an obsession.

Even with my prescription, and seemingly blissful life since I began my medication, I can't shake the belt obsession. My tools, however, are not always easily found because I can't remember where they are anymore. My belts, otherwise, are either around my waist or hanging in my closet.

The Mind is a Filing Cabinet

OCD "is a gift and a curse" as stated by the TV detective, "Monk." We not only notice everything, but we can remember almost everything. It is not photographic memory, and it did me no good in college on tests. The memories are usually instances I would rather forget. Since OCD is a curse, however, I was able to tag certain memories with reminders, akin to placing sticky notes to mark the pages of a textbook.

Certain songs, TV shows, sounds, smells and visions remind me of situations I'd rather forget. In the moment a bad experience actually occurred, I would say to myself, "I will always think of that experience when I hear a particular sound." Now, every time I hear that sound, that awful memory comes rushing back.

I also never had to write anything down. I would always remember dates, times and places where I was supposed to be. The anxiety of missing those dates was too great, and many times they would haunt me throughout the day and night, and I would constantly check my watch, clock or calendar to ensure I would not miss an appointment.

As a child, lying in my bed at home in one of my twin beds, I could see the red-lighted digital clock on my desk. When waking in the middle of the night, it is always good to know the time so you know how much longer you have to sleep.

One of the strangest games my mind ever played on me involved this digital clock. Two different times brought two unique situations: 3:15 a.m. and 11:11 p.m.

Since my home was in the eastern-standard time zone, and the movie of the week came on at 9:00 and ended at 11:00, I would sometimes get to bed just after 11:00. Since this ritual was a time ritual, I would have to wait on the clock. As the clock ticked and finally landed on the time 11:11, I would have to say, in this order, every night, "Eleven-eleven, eleven past eleven, one thousand one hundred eleven, one hundred eleven point one, eleven point eleven, one point one hundred eleven, point one thousand one hundred eleven, eleven-eleven."

The freakier part came later in the darkest part of the night, and it all stems from a book called the *Amityville Horror*. In this book, all members of the family who had previously lived in the haunted house being portrayed, were all killed at the precise time of 3:15 a.m. I had read far enough into the book to extract that information before putting it down for good. From that point forward for many years, when I would wake up in the middle of the night, the time on my clock would always be 3:15. I would absolutely freak!

Since the ritual required me to look at the clock, I could

not just turn over and close my eyes. If I did, I would not be able to go back to sleep. I would lie awake, without looking at the clock sometimes for 20 minutes, hoping the haunted time would have passed. After feeling like I had waited long enough, I would complete the ritual by looking at the clock, and it would inevitably read, "3:15." "OH, NO!" I have no idea how my body clock played this trick on me, but it did and it scared the shit out of me. Then, I would really have a hard time going back to sleep.

OCD and My Job

When I was in college, and in my first working days as a professional, I worked for a carpet manufacturer. Hailing from Georgia, that was not an uncommon occupation. The job actually offered some pretty spectacular opportunities in that I traveled all over the world selling and maintaining carpet installations.

In the early years, I did mostly repair work on installations either badly installed or manufactured with a flaw, the most common one called a "trailing edge." This meant, at the seam, there was excess yarn sticking up which needed to be trimmed manually with a pair of carpet scissors. Sounds easy, except this was carpet tile, so this seam appeared every eighteen inches. We did some big jobs eighteen inches at a time, and the Atlanta Hartsfield International Airport concourses was one of them.

Two very particular jobs come to mind where OCD resulted in less-than-desired outcomes. The first was in Houston at a very large installation of 30,000 square yards.

Since it was so large and there were only two people on site with two pair of scissors, it could not possibly get done in a timely manner. Moreover, our jeans and shoes would wear out while crawling on the floor and our thumbs would become completely numb and unusable by the week's end.

My boss was a tinkerer and inventor of machines, and he built an electric machine with a rotary blade. The object was to push the machine down the seam, cutting the excess yarn making the pile all the same level. He sent one of his flunkies to Houston to test it and show us how to use it. The machine was about the size of a circular saw and spun its blade just as fast. Depending on the height of the carpet, the blade could be adjusted to get the best cut, but we had to unplug the machine to make the adjustments because there was no "on-off" switch. When it was plugged in, it was on.

While we were testing the machine, the enormous responsibility of plugging and unplugging the machine between adjustments was given to me. The man had no idea he had given this task to someone with an extreme mental disorder, nor did he know his fingers were at risk of getting chopped off.

At one point he asked me to unplug the machine so he could make an adjustment. I unplugged it, and in the instant I heard the machine stop, OCD made me put the plug back into the outlet. I do not remember what the consequence would have been had I not performed the ritual, but whatever it was it could have been worth the cost of that guy loosing his fingers. No matter though, because in the small amount of time between unplugging the machine and re-plugging it, I decided the made-up consequence was of greater evil than the chance of someone losing a limb – albeit a small limb.

After placing the plug back in the outlet, I immediately unplugged it and turned to face the man who was handling the machine. He gave me the look you would expect, and I just pretended that it was an accident (I did not mean to stick it back into the outlet. It just happened). I really thought he would buy that? Lucky for me, no fingers were lost and no blood was let. My OCD survived another incident with no harm to anyone.

We used the machine for another couple of tries, and then went back to completing the 30,000 square yard, two-week trimming job with scissors.

The next job was with Northwest Airlines in Minneapolis. It is a nice place in the summertime, and the women there are beautiful. Given some free time up there, I would probably have had a good time. Of course, I did have some free time there, but my OCD stole it from me. It was another trim job of 10,000 square yards. Two other trimmers and I were sent to do the work, and it was tedious as usual.

After spending our first night out at the nightclub owned by the artist formerly known as Prince, we figured there had to be something else to this town besides that over the top, crazy, weird place. The only thing I could wonder about the people who were there was what they could possibly do with themselves when it was light outside. The patrons were all dressed in black and covered with body piercings and tattoos. The three of us were dressed in jeans and polo shirts, and we were way out of place. There was also this family of three there. The parents must have taken their daughter (she was obviously not of admission age) to see the pop rocker's bar. They were really out of place, and the young lady looked kind of embarrassed for talking her parents into bringing her there. Her parents just looked puzzled.

Back at work the next day, our job carried on as usual until our foreman arrived. He seemed to take the position that doing this job was not necessary. I figured it did not fit into his schedule and that he just wanted to go back home. The other guy with us had a date in Minneapolis that night (and a girlfriend back home) so he quickly agreed that leaving town first thing in the morning was a good idea. The third grunt and I said we needed to finish the job we were sent to do, but we were overruled and left the job site.

Most common laborers like me would have agreed with the person in charge and headed on home, but neither I, nor the third grunt, would have any part of it. We decided to take matters into our own hands and arrange with a security guard in the building to let us back in around midnight. It was like dumb following dumber, with me being the latter, of course.

I had a fraternity brother living in Minneapolis at the time, and he took my fellow snipper and me out to dinner and to a bar full of gorgeous ladies. I could not believe my eyes. I thought women this nice looking only existed in the South. Before we knew it, it was midnight and the guard was expecting us. To this day, I can't believe we left to do something that would hold no pleasant memory for the future. As the OCD rule goes, we did not do it because we wanted to;

we did it because we had to. We had to do it to finish the job, to do good by the people who sent us, so to not look bad, to satisfy our conscious (in my case, an obsession), to not get fired... I was 22 years old, for crying out loud, and fun was to be had, but I left anyway to go trim carpet tiles at midnight.

Our reward did come later. A few weeks following our return, we were scheduled to fly out to do another job in some awful place like Cincinnati or Sioux City. The other two were ironically sent back to Minneapolis to finish the Northwestern job. We were told the customer had much better results when the OCDer was up there working. Some reward. The lazy snippers got to go back, and we were sent to a second tier job where the ladies were not nearly as good looking.

The Fire at Nike

After I graduated from college, I was given the most amazing opportunity to travel to Australia and work for two years selling carpet tiles to commercial properties. I blended right in with the culture and became a player in business and social circles. It was the absolute time of my life, but OCD followed me there to disrupt what could have been an absolutely perfect life.

Upon hearing on Australian TV that some boy was looking for a bone marrow transplant, I obsessed that I was the one with the match he needed and should call the TV station and let them know. I fought the obsession, but with difficulty, because this situation did involve a life. Was I a match? I don't know, but surely the professionals had ways of finding someone who was. There was no announcement on the TV giving the blood type and no number to call if a viewer could help. But the thing that helped me overcome the obsession was knowing that every other viewer watching the same show only saw it for what it was, just a TV show. When other viewers clicked the channel or turned it off, they surely went about their normal lives without a worry.

Following my years in Sydney, my boss wanted me to move to Singapore. I declined at first, but I truly loved my company and the mentor who helped me to conquer Australia. I decided to go, but this time I would be working with a completely different product. A flooring product still, but this one was a raised flooring system under which wires could run. It was a perfect fit for our company because once installed, we could sell them the carpet to go on top.

Somewhere along the way in my training, I heard the pedestals on which the flooring sat on top would melt in a fire. The pedestals were only a couple of inches high, but this became an obsession that would hamper my success as a salesperson and change the product forever.

When first learning of the problem, I pictured people trying to run out of a burning building and not making it out because they would sink into a melting floor. A friend of mine told me not to worry about that because once those pedestals caught fire, the people would die of asphyxiation before having the chance to escape. I thought, "You know, he is right, so I should not worry about people melting into the floor." After a short while of taking comfort in the asphyxiation theory, I returned to the floor-melting obsession.

With every person with whom I trained before leaving for Asia, I would bring up the issue of fire. They all looked at me like it was a non-issue and moved on to something else. I carried that obsession from Kansas City to a strip club in Montreal and into a classroom to learn everything about the product. I asked sensible questions attempting to mask my obsessions, but every other question I asked was regarding flammability.

On my way to Singapore, I stopped over in Paris to complete my training. The product was invented in France, so I was sure to get the straight answer there. After presenting the question more than once to a salesperson and to some people in the manufacturing plant, they all told me it was a non-issue and not to worry about it. The bottom line here was the obsession was so strong that no matter what people said to assure me it was okay as is, in my mind I could still vision people trying to get out of a burning building where this stuff was installed.

My first installation of this product was in a Nike office in Jakarta on the island of Java in Indonesia. The experience with the local installers was like none other in my life – total confusion. I asked for a chalk line, a band saw and screw drill. What I got was a box of chalk, a hacksaw and a screwdriver. Then the workers wanted to load up all the steel decking and take it across town to a machine shop somewhere in Jakarta. That is when the nightmare and what I thought to be a great omen struck: the fire alarm in the 50-story building went off. We all had to evacuate through the stairwells some thirty stories to the outside. Even though the installation we were completing was just in a small computer room, I knew this was a sign of things to come, and that there was no way in hell I should be selling this "dangerous" product.

With all the positives going on around me – a beautiful blue sky, Indonesians squatting around me, smoking, talking and laughing, the promise of a fun night out with some locals and my boss, the enjoyment of being able to communicate with people who spoke no word of English and I no word of Indonesian – I only sat there in a cloud of dread that what I was doing was going to cost lives.

The fire alarm stopped because nothing was really on fire, and we went back upstairs to continue the work. I realized then that the moment of destruction on one of my installations might not happen for years. I would possibly be in a new career back in the States and hear of a catastrophic fire in Jakarta and I would be responsible for all the deaths that occurred. I could see myself elsewhere in the world having a normal life, but all would come crashing down when the inevitable happened. The devastation would be my fault, and I would not only have to live with it but would have to return to Indonesia and surrender myself to authorities. My family would be left behind, but my obsession of returning to admit to selling a product I knew to be dangerous would have to be satisfied.

There were no rituals I could perform to keep all of that from happening. I had to do what was necessary to keep that product, in its current makeup, from ever being installed in any building under my watch.

Upon returning to Singapore, I started to hint to my boss that I thought the product was no good. He agreed, but this man opened up all of Asia for the company and sold more carpet than anyone I ever knew. He also had a firm belief that carpet was nasty as hell and he would never have it in his own home. He felt, as I should have felt: Go out and sell the stuff. It is good enough, and if the higher-ups in the company thought it bad, we would not be selling it. "End of story," it should have been, and I should have listened and moved on.

While most people do not do research into government regulations to try and find the one that will disrupt the progress of their own business, I set out to find the one roadblock that would run my business into a wall. After meeting with a fire official who was knowledgeable of the British Standards for building materials, I found the needed roadblock to relieve me of my obsession.

Since most of Asia at one time had been under British Colonial rule, or under the rule of some European nation, most of Asia abided by building standards established by the British. The fire official told me that if my product did not meet certain criteria such as weight load, impact load, combustion, oxygen depletion... it would not be able to be sold in much of Asia. Note, none of the tests he mentioned had anything to do with melting, but remember OCD is not reality, and my obsession still had to do with people unable to escape a fire because they could not walk out of a building without sinking into the floor. Whether any of the tests determined melting to be a hazard, it did not matter. My mind was already made up that it was a hazard.

My next move was to schedule testing of the product by the Singapore Institute of Building Standards. It seemed everything in Singapore was named the "Singapore Institute" of something. Testing was arranged, and I sat by praying the product would not meet standards. My OCD forced me to root against something that could make me a lot of money and push my reputation as a successful international businessman to an even higher level. I was like a double agent: someone working for the good of the company while at the same time trying to destroy it from within. I was a mole, and no one would be the beneficiary of this long-drawn out ritual created to prevent the fabricated consequence.

When the results came in, I was elated! The tests showed the product met every other standard except combustion and oxygen depletion. The product could not be sold where British Standards applied!

However, I kept my job and helped develop a steel structure to replace the plastic pedestals. To this very day, the steel is used rather than the plastic for this product, but I ultimately was unsuccessful in my attempt to sell a large quantity of the product because the manufacturing costs at that time were too high.

Abbott Labs

After receiving my first container-load of steel product, I was in competition with three other companies in a bid to install raised flooring in an office space. We were all asked to present our products at the same time to the customer. It was very unusual to make a presentation in front of the customer and your competition at the same time!

The customer was Abbott Laboratories, and they were a huge multinational company. For me to win this job would be a great first step for the new product and work nicely as a showcase to other potential clients.

Amazingly, with the highest price, I won the job. With the product already in Singapore, it was installed quickly and just in time for me to brag about it at my upcoming sales meeting in Australia.

For my presentation, I needed pictures of the product actually installed. I had plenty of other pictures to show how it worked and what it looked like in sample and mock-up installations, but none of it in a real, workable setting. When I got to Australia, I still did not have a picture of it. It was not because I did not take any pictures. I had taken plenty of the installation at Abbott, but had destroyed them all before my meeting by ripping them to shreds and throwing them away.

After the installation was complete, I went back to Abbott Labs to take pictures. Upon entering the complex, I reread a sign I had passed by many times during my work at the office site, "No pagers, cell phones or cameras allowed beyond this point. Electronic devices may spark fires." My camera was well hidden in my pocket, so the security guard did not stop me. After snapping the pictures, I left with the satisfaction of not being caught and not setting any fires.

With the photos developed and sitting on my desk at the

office, I became obsessed with what that sign read and wondered if my camera had made a spark and did start a fire. The unbelievable scenario actually crossed my mind that there could be a delayed reaction, and perhaps my camera's electronic signal could still be in the Abbott complex and had not yet relinquished its ability to cause a spark and a fire. Obsessions made me believe in impossible consequences, but this one was more than ridiculous.

No matter how stupid this all seemed, I obsessed that the whole of Abbott Laboratories Singapore, Ltd. was going to burn to the ground, and it would be my fault. Ironically, after all I had done to get the product to meet fire codes so as not to worry about people and property being burned to a crisp, I obsessed that me taking a picture would have the same result.

I had to destroy my photographic evidence so the police could not connect me to this disaster surely to take place. In the end, there was no picture, no showcase, no bragging rights, and no fire.

The Things That Could Happen

OCD looks into the future and fabricates consequences. Not only do I make things up that could happen from fictitious arrangements and imaginary sequences, but I can create possible consequences from actions and objects that actually exist.

One such occasion was in my backyard in New Orleans. I suddenly had a fascination of cutting down small trees and overhanging limbs. I borrowed one of those telescoping tree pruners from my neighbor and commenced to lop everything in site. At the end of a pruner, there is a cutting device that works by trapping a limb in a void and then pulling a rope activating a spring-loaded blade to cut the limb. There is also a curved saw with very sharp teeth for cutting larger limbs opposite the spring blade. My backyard was only 40 X 60 feet, and there was a small hazard going right down the middle of it – the main power line to my house.

As I was swung the blade violently in the air cutting

down any branch in the path of my blade, a freshly cut limb caught itself on the power line. I enthusiastically reached the blade up to the wire to release the stuck limb, but suddenly I froze. I stared at the electricity source and slowly backed off, dropping the pruner. Through the front gate I went, and to the front porch I sat with my head in my hands. My sweaty palms felt clammy to my forehead and with that feeling came a head-rush, dizziness and nausea. I thought I should be dead.

I pictured the paramedics bringing me from the backyard in a black-plastic bag on their way to the coroner's black station wagon. My wife and my neighbors were crowded around watching, and thinking, "He should have known better." For any normal person, the sight of the power line may have simply put an end to their work. For me, however, anxiety was my punishment, and it stuck with me for days.

The Peanut

As I made sales calls one day, a peanut found its way from a peanut jar I was snacking from to between my legs on the car seat. While parked under the awning of a condominium, and without even thinking, I tossed the peanut from my car into the parking lot. As I left my car to complete a delivery of tourist magazines to a beach resort, I pictured a small child being placed on the pavement as a vacationer unloaded luggage. I pictured the child picking up the peanut, placing it in its mouth and choking to death on it. Back at the car, I frantically searched the brick driveway for the nut, and picked it up. The worst part about this obsession was that it occurred even after I had been on the OCD suppressant Zoloft, at 200 milligrams a day, for 10 years.

At my next stop, I threw the peanut safely into some bushes and made my next delivery. But in my mind, I created a similar scene, except this time, the child crawled from the pavement into the bushes, found the peanut hidden in the pine straw, swallowed it and choked to death. I crawled into the bushes, searched the ground cover, found the peanut and threw it back into the car. To the best of my knowledge, the peanut is still somewhere in my car.

The Damaged Tire

In another instance, just off Georgia Hwy. 27, on the road to my father's house, I noticed the car in front of me had an imperfection on one of its tires. A white patch was appearing and disappearing as the car rolled forward. I had to follow this car to let the driver and passenger know a hazard may lead to a really bad accident if they did not do something about their tire. I pictured tomorrow's newspaper headline: "Two people killed in car accident." The sub-heading read, "Faulty tire suspected."

I followed the car to a nearby parking lot where they came to a stop. No matter what my schedule may have been, I felt it a lifesaving duty to stop them as they walked toward a store. Politely, they told me the white patch was on the tire because it was brand new, and it was probably the bar-code sticker. A few more miles, and the sticker would have been gone.

The Log and the Trucker

On a long, lonely, stretch of highway between Jackson, MS and New Orleans, I got behind a log truck. I noticed as it bounced along the interstate, a log was balanced like a pencil on a finger. With every imperfection in the roadway, it teetered like a seesaw with its fulcrum a single chain in the middle of the trailer. I could see the headlines in the McComb, MS fish wrapper, "Driver killed by log dislodged from truck." So I stayed behind the truck studying the log and its balancing act, apparently not believing I could be the person referred to in tomorrow's headline. Other cars kept passing me without concern for the log or its future victim.

Sometimes the law of physics, and just plain reality, are ignored by a mind plagued with OCD. I should reword the beginning of that last sentence to read, "Most of the time," or "All of the time." If a log drops from a truck going 65mph, the log will not at first come to a complete stop and go through someone's windshield. The driver of the car behind should have enough time to avoid the log as it skids down the highway. The reality of the situation would be that if I were to somehow flag down the trucker and have him pull over so I may show him the potential problem, tomorrow's headline would read, "Trucker Kills Paranoid Traveler."

On one occasion, I actually followed a trucker to a truck stop to inform him he had a blown-out tire on his trailer. This was an 18-wheeler and he had 17 other good tires, but I was worried someone might get hurt. At 9:00 at night the sparks coming off the bare wheel made quite a spectacle, and made it look all the more dangerous. The trucker said nothing and only smiled. He must have thought, "What an idiot, and hell if I am buying a new $300 tire on this $600 delivery."

Air Travel

Whenever traveling by airplane, I hate sitting in a wing seat. The responsibility is too great, and not the responsibility given by the crew of opening up the emergency door in case of the need to escape. No, the responsibility comes with watching the wing, and making sure it stays together. All of those rivets holding the wing together are my responsibility. Making sure there is no leaking hydraulic fluid is also a concern along with any icy build-up that may occur. The headline could read, "Cautious passenger saves hundreds from certain peril." It would really go something like this, "Oh stewardess, would you please climb over the other two people in my row, look out the window and check the 14th rivet there. I believe it is coming loose." Headline reads, "Passenger thrown from aircraft through the emergency exit at "28,000 feet." Sub-heading would read, "Crew and passengers offer no comments."

The Sand Pit

There is nothing like walking hand-in-hand with the one you love on a nice secluded beach in the fall season. The air is cool and there is usually good surf, and you can still walk barefoot on the Northwest Florida beaches without getting cold.

It is a scene offering pure relaxation for normal people, but pure agony for me. While walking by a group of adults and children digging a large sand pit, I could only flash back to an article reporting the death of a child who suffocated because the hole he was digging himself into collapsed around him. The incident had recently happened on the same beach upon which we were walking.

The article did not detail the type of hole he dug but logic would assume it would have been fairly narrow and deep. The hole presently dug on the beach in front of us was more of a crater and posed no danger to the people digging it. As a side note, they were also having a great time with their little construction project.

My fiancé was talking away, and probably saying something important, but I heard not a word. I was only focused on those people sinking into the sand and suffocating. I had to make a plan of attack to pause or walk and go back to warn the fun-loving family. After explaining the article to my walking partner, she seemed to understand, so I walked back down the beach and explained to one of the adults the dangerous act they were committing, and subjecting their children to such an activity could result in their death. Talk about a fun sponge! Oh, I referred to the article and the recent tragedy, and that made *me* feel the warning to be credible. In reality, however, I knew the hole they were digging was too wide to collapse.

The obsession of someone else suffocating in the sand because it could happen, and had recently happened, was all too great for me to overcome. I was never concerned about the welfare of any of those people, but only for my own conscious because if anyone of those people had suffocated, it would have been my fault!

To further show how strong this obsession was, there was a topless lady sunbathing just down the beach from the hole and I chose not to stare at her instead. Looking back, I can't believe I turned around. However, I must admit, at this point in my relationship, I had not yet mastered the skill of being able to stare at a pretty lady without my future wife noticing.

The Coat-Hanger Monkey

Living in Singapore was kind of like living on a college campus. Everything was so institutionalized; you had to go outside the campus grounds (in this case, the country) to find real fun. When stuck on campus, or in Singapore, you had to really create fun.

On most weekends, a trip across the bridge to Malaysia or a boat ride to Indonesia brought good times, but budgets and time did not always allow for such trips, so we had to make the best of it on the island. A couple of friends and I decided to climb the ever intimidating highest point in Singapore – Bukit Timah. It is a whopping 573 feet high and has a paved road all the way to the top. Bukit Timah is also a significant landmark because it survived the bulldozing of most high areas during the island's man-made expansion into the sea.

Atop the mountain there are a couple of quarries, some jungle and wild monkeys. They could also be called urban monkeys, because they are pretty much isolated having to live their lives in this small wilderness amongst the concrete towers. While admiring our surroundings, a group of monkeys appeared before us, and we took pictures and taunted them. For the most part, they were fun and acted in good spirits. There was, however, this one monkey with a coat hanger around its waist. It kept beating on it and pulling at it, but it was not coming lose. It had been around the monkey's waist for quite sometime, because its skin had grown around parts of it, and the wire was obviously cutting into its insides. The image became seared into my mind, and with OCD there was no letting go of it.

For weeks, I thought of calling someone about it. Having no idea who to call, the Singapore Institution of Something or the Other, I just dwelled on the sight of that poor monkey and thought of the pain it must feel. The obsession led me to dream up the conversation I would have with this institute. After I told them about the monkey, they would say, "Oh, you mean Ol' Coat-Hanger Monkey. We know all about him. He is impossible to catch, but sweet as Durian. Thank you for calling us, but it is really out of our hands."

After playing that conversation over and over again in my head, I lied to myself that that is certainly what they would really say. I doubt it, and that monkey probably suffered, but sometimes obsessions confuse one's understanding of real and fantasy. Was I obsessed about this monkey because I really cared, or was I obsessed about this monkey because it was only my mind creating this obsession?

Unfortunately, during my life, I have had to ask the

question of whether I really cared about the outcome of an event, or has my mind fooled me into *thinking* that I cared. The question is never really answered, because so many times OCD has forced me to question my own sincerity.

The Oven and the Stove

Losing your house to fire is probably the worst thing that could happen next to losing your health. Fortunately, for me, I have lost neither so I only make that assumption based on personal theory.

When I obsess about leaving my stove or oven on, I picture my house burning to the ground. To prevent losing my house I would return home and ensure the appliance in question is turned off. The result would be that my house would be saved. The difficulty in this obsession is that turning an appliance off to prevent the house from burning down is a reasonable action. I am not obsessing about a disease that I could alone prevent. That would be a fantasy and the ritual to prevent the consequence of disease is usually quite convenient (shooting birds at myself or saying "shit head" twice...). My house burning down to the ground, however, is something that could actually happen if I had left the stove or oven on.

The only ritual that could satisfy the oven or stove obsession is to actually perform the physical requirement of switching the appliance off. That means, wherever I happen to be, I must relocate myself to the location of the object of obsession to perform the ritual, or have someone else perform the ritual for me.

One such instance occurred on a trip home to New Orleans from a rental I had in Florida. I was thirty minutes into the trip before I talked myself into believing I had left the stove on. My kitchen was an afterthought to the design of my garage apartment, so it was very small and crammed into a tiny area. The paper towel rack hung just above the stove making it the perfect fuel for a fire.

I tried to talk myself out of it, but thought if I really did leave it on, my computer and other items would be destroyed. Since my belongings were in danger it made sense to go back just to make sure. I turned the car around and made the trip back costing me an hour of precious time. The odd thing about this kind of obsession is that I never really get upset and pound the steering wheel and yell, because if I really did leave an appliance on that could cause a fire, then turning back to prevent a disaster is worth it. The anxiety happens when the thoughts occur, but once knowing this thing that could happen is reality and not fantasy, then I have no choice but to perform the ritual.

While skiing out in Colorado, I obsessed about leaving some wet socks on a heating radiator at a friend's house. I pictured her little mountain home burning to the ground and it being my entire fault. As I was up on a mountain, I called my hostess to let her know of my dilemma. She had to leave work to check on the situation, and sure enough my socks were on the radiator.

There was a one out of 100 chance that obsession was actually reality. Unfortunately, for those with OCD, obsessions involving something that could happen have the real possibility of occurring if the ritual of returning to the location is not performed.

A Financial Risk

Obsessions also could cost a lot of money, especially if they are unwarranted like most obsessions are.

Parallel Parking

After moving to Australia, I immediately began looking for a place to live. My boss planned to help me when he got to town, but I could not wait. After I asked the young lady at my hotel's front desk where someone my age might like to live, I left with the classifieds advertising places to rent and began my search on a nasty, rainy day. I had only been in the country for a few days, and my driving was a bit erratic since I was not used to driving on the left side of the road. I also had a cold and, with a weakening voice and a cowboy hat upon my head, must have seemed a quite unattractive prospect for a "wanted flatmate."

Cars and real estate are expensive in Australia. I never really understood why, but property was a coveted and asset. The place to live for people around my age of 24 was in the

North Sydney area just above Sydney Harbor. Parking was limited in the area, so parallel parking was common. I consider myself one of the greatest parallel parkers in the United States, but this was a whole new ballgame driving on the right-hand side of the car. At one residence, I backed into my spot successfully but bumped the car behind me. Having this happen is not unusual and, for just this reason, cars do have bumpers. Most drivers whose car "just kisses" the one behind in a parallel park maneuver think only of it as a way of making sure the car fits. Not me, though.

The car I bumper-kissed was a nice little sports car. Once my car came to a stop between the sports car and the one in front of me, I went back to inspect the bumper I hit. There was a nice little dent in the fender of the car I could not have possibly created. I thought about it a minute, then went up to the flat to meet my new potential roommate.

Instead of me just checking the place out for my consideration, I found myself being interviewed by the current tenant and then shown around the apartment. This procedure was like going through fraternity rush as a freshman at Auburn University. When I left, they would say something to the effect, "Don't call us, we will call you."

Back at my car, I inspected the wound on the fender of the sports car, again. Once convincing myself I had not made that dent, I drove away. The obsession then became that I had damaged someone's property and my being dishonest about it was a terrible thing. Guilt and anxiety soon followed, and the only thing I could do to reverse the guilt was to drive back to the car and leave a note on the windshield.

Adding anymore drive time to my day was stupid enough, but leaving a note on that car was even dumber. If the driver of that sports car was dishonest, he could have dialed my work number and taken me up on my claim of being responsible for hitting his car. Thank goodness he did not. If he had, I would not have been able to forgive myself for throwing good money away to fix something I did not damage. As a person with OCD, I did not recognize expensive consequences as a deterrent to satisfy an obsession.

I went to four places that day, with one showing me the "toilet" instead of the bathroom, another wiping from his leather couch the ink that had spilled from the broken pen in my back pocket, and another giving me a shocked look when I said, "I'll take it!" None of those people called me. The fourth one did call me to let me know I could move in with them and thank you God that they did, because they were the ones that were to become not only life-long friends, but also my supporting cast for my "at least three things a day" obsession.

Shoes by the Door

Singapore was another one of my overseas residences, and with it came the custom of leaving your shoes at the front door. I had just moved into my British "Black and White" home when my new roommates decided to have a number of people over for a social gathering. For each person who attended, there were two shoes left by the front door.

With my fiancé back in the United States, I wanted to

send to her photos of what life was like on the equator and what she was to expect upon her arrival. With my camera in hand, I took a photo of the shoes. I took another, and another, and, still, another. These photographs were taken with a camera using film. Back in the 20th century, digital cameras were yet to be invented and the cost of taking pictures was two-fold: having to buy the film and then having to develop the pictures. There was also no choice on which ones were to be developed. When turning in a roll to the camera store, all photos were developed and, no matter whether they turned out or not, payment was expected.

Knowing this financial burden, I continued to snap pictures of the shoes until reaching the number eight on a 24-frame roll of film. Because I obsessed with getting different angles of the shot, one-third of my roll was wasted. Looking on the bright side, at least the technology of the electric flash had been invented, and I had not wasted any flashcubes.

The Hanging Limb

In the year 1995, Hurricane Erin blew through Northwest Florida as a category 1 storm. I sat in my father-in-law's house with my wife and him watching out the window as Erin made a direct hit on Pensacola. This was my first hurricane to witness first hand and, because it was a weak one, my safety was never in danger.

The wind was a steady 80 mph for an hour from one direction and then for an hour in the other direction once the eye passed over. During the first hour, trees cracked and fell in the streets and large limbs from those that did not fall either made their way to the ground or hung on for dear life on what was left of the tree from which they fell.

My car was parked in the road just in front of the house, and it was fascinating to watch the rain blow around it. I could see the car's aerodynamic engineering at work, and it looked like it was in one of those wind tunnels seen in car commercials.

During the first half of the storm, a large limb hanging by a thread above my car was swinging just above its beautiful paint job. Should it let go, there would be probably just enough damage for me only to meet my insurance deductible. I would have liked to venture outside and either moved my car or pulled the limb down. However, with the wind blowing 80 mph, I figured that would not be such a good idea.

After the first hour of fury passed, the eye of the storm surrounded the house. The sun came out, and the wind died. The sound of chainsaws began to fire up and people came outside of their houses to assess property damage or clean up what they could before the other side of the storm hit.

The eye of a storm seemingly offers the same opportunity two fighting armies may give each other to clear the battlefield of their dead and wounded. Once the allotted time is up, however, the fighting begins just as fierce as it was prior to the ceasefire.

Here was my opportunity to grab the tree limb from its threatening position above my car. I stood there, not moving and only watching. I have heard that some of the worst injuries from hurricanes do not occur during the actual storm, but in the cleanup. People may step on live wires resulting in electrocution, cut their arms off with their own chain saws, fall from ladders while attempting to clean their roofs, have a heart attack from overworking... All these things you read about in the paper such as, "Joe Doe made it through the storm only to die from a chain saw his neighbor dropped on him while he was holding his buddy's ladder. The saw only grazed his arm, but at the sight of it coming down he had a heart attack. As he grabbed his chest and fell backwards, he fell on a live wire and was electrocuted."

I stood on the front porch obsessing over becoming a victim of an "eye of the storm" injury. I made myself believe that if I were to walk 40 feet to my car to knock the potential $500 deductible-meeting tree limb to the ground that I would become a statistic. I obsessed that my new wife would lose me if one of those hard-green pinecones fell from 50 feet above and split my head wide open. The anxiety was enough to keep me from going outside to remove the limb. I could actually hear people saying, "He should have known better than to go out there and risk his life for the sake of possibly saving $500."

For the next hour, I sat by the window anxiously watching that limb swing over my car while 80 mph winds blew in the opposite direction as before.

When the storm ended, I walked out, moved the car, and pulled down the limb. I obsessed that going out there during the eye of the storm was more dangerous than waiting until after the storm. The consequence of me going against the ritual of staying indoors would have been a well-publicized death or injury. The real consequence of me going out there would have been the logical removal of the limb. One thing about OCD is that it never works in a logical manner.

US Postal Service

After I left my multinational sales manager position in Singapore, the home office in Atlanta promised me a choice of four different positions I could fill once back in the United States. I never found out what those positions were, and the company quit sending me paychecks about six months after my move back home. Suddenly, I was unemployed. During those six months, of which one of my friends referred to as "the salad days," I had also been looking for other employment but had found none.

Unemployment is a dreadful position to find yourself. Waking up in the morning and helping your wife get off to work is a humbling experience. Once she drove away, I would spend my entire day looking for a job and have no fun during the hunt. Any fun I may have had would be followed with guilt because one should not have fun while one's wife is the breadwinner.

I could spend no money and had to save what little I did have. Any errand I ran, I usually walked to my destination. My trips were usually to the bank to withdraw from our savings, or to the post office to mail resumes. The post office is a great place to go when you are bored, because you feel like you are getting something done, even if it is only to drop a letter or buy a first-class stamp. I found a lot of other people felt the same way because there were always many retirees standing in line with me. There was also a homeless guy who was always busy filling out postal forms found in those little pigeonholes where the little pens are chained to the countertops. (Sometimes those pens actually work!)

I finally took a part-time job at a store as a work-boot salesperson for just over minimum wage. One day, two rednecks came in to buy some boots. The one who was being fit for a new pair had a snuff-stuffed lower lip, and the other stood around with his hands in his pockets. After trying on about three pair, Snuff Lip looked over to his friend and said, "Hey Bubba, run out to the truck and get my spit cup. I'm about to drown." After forcing myself to keep down my lunch, I could only think, "Six years of college and four years of international business experience down the drain."

Every penny I made from working at that shoe store was earned, and I was even more careful with the money I spent, or so I thought.

One day, I must have received a pretty fancy rejection letter in the mail, because the enclosure was in an oversized manila envelope. There were four first-class postage stamps on the top-right side of the envelope, and they were clean. They had no postmark stamped across them, so they could be used again! They were worth about 15 minutes worth of work at my just-above-minimum-wage job, and any 15 minutes fitting rednecks with boots was a long time.

I cut the stamps away from the envelope, and tossed the

envelope in the trash. I went to my desk and placed the stamps in the top right-hand drawer with my other mailing materials. Then I thought of the people who worked at the post office, of the lines of bored customers who were maybe going to spend only what's required of them to buy a single stamp, and of the homeless guy who wasted form after form of postal material. I thought of the postman delivering mail to remote areas where it was impossible for a profit to be made from a single stamp on that kind of delivery.

I took the stamps out of my drawer and threw them away. I walked back to my desk with my head in my hands and thought how stupid this was. I just threw away the equivalent of a sum greater than one dollar. I retrieved the stamps from the trashcan once again.

After rethinking the moral obligation I had to the USPS (which was none) and of all those lives affected should I make use of those stamps, I took a pair of scissors and cut the stamps in half and threw them away. I yelled at myself for this stupid action, but I could not kill the obsession that by reusing these stamps I would be immoral in the eyes of God. These stamps may well have been a small gift from God offering a glimmer of light in an otherwise gloomy day. Looking back on all of my other obsessions, I wonder how many other small gifts from God may have been overlooked.

At the end of the day, I overcame two obsessions by destroying the stamps: one being the risk of being immoral and the other an obsession that was wasting valuable time. If I had not cut those stamps in half, many trips would have been made back and fourth to the trashcan retrieving and then throwing away those stupid stamps. However, the anxiety of it all clearly was not worth the 15 minutes it would take to sell a pair of boots to a couple of rednecks.

The Passport and Plane Tickets

During my life, I have traveled to 35 US states, three Canadian provinces, lived in four different countries (five counting Louisiana) and traveled to 15 others in Europe, Asia, the South Pacific and Central America. When traveling by air, all you really need is a passport or state approved ID and your plane ticket. Everything else can be purchased at your destination. Although, to make things easier, let's include a wallet, some money and a credit card as necessities.

I like to travel, but my preparation is stressful and exhausting. The night before a trip begins, I usually stay up late packing clothes and personals in a large bag (usually involves doing laundry and searching frantically for that one piece of clothing necessary for the trip). I usually lay all articles of clothing on the bed, and make sure the number of outfits matches the number of days I will be away.

The next bag is the easiest to pack, but the most difficult to travel with. It is my backpack/carry on. In this bag are a book, diary and pen for writing about the trip, extra contacts for the eyes, a comb, travel guide, camera, passport and airline tickets. The latter two are the most important. This bag will never leave my side, and should never leave my shoulder (but sometimes it does).

The problem with this bag is the objects within it have the ability to hop out and run around, and possibly disappear forever. For this reason, I have to check, before I turn out my light, that my plane ticket and passport are in my bag. After my light is out, I lay there wondering if they may have fallen out while I was checking to see if they were in there, so I turn my light back on to check again. When I zip my bag closed, I make sure to watch the objects disappear behind the zipper.

The next morning, before leaving the house, I look into my bag to ensure once again they are in my bag. After placing my bags in the trunk of my car, I check once again. This is the least stressful check, because I know if they escape the bag during the trip, they will only go as far as the trunk is big.

Cruising down the highway, anxiety sets in and I begin to think that perhaps neither object was in my bag, and that I will get to the airport and have not a ticket or passport. Arguably, they are in the bag and the bag is in the trunk. I saw them with my own eyes, so I need to relax and drive on.

"Damn it." They may have fallen on the bumper and out of the car when I last checked.

"They did not!" My hands grip the steering wheel tighter, and I tense up while continuing the drive.

"Just think, though, how much more at ease I would be just knowing for sure." I pull the car into the emergency lane of the interstate, get out of the car and go to the trunk. After unzipping the bag, I see both articles safely sitting in my bag.

As cars whiz by me at 75 or 80 mph, I run back to the driver's side of the car and toss my bag on the passenger seat. Now it is where I can keep an eye on it. Before pulling out into traffic, I unzip the bag to make sure neither article dropped out between the trunk and the passenger seat. Nope, they are both there.

After arriving at the airport and parking my car, and locking it three times and pulling on the handle to make for damn sure it is locked, I proceed to check-in. I have in my left hand the big bag, my backpack thrown over my shoulder, and in my right hand is my ticket and passport. They now will not leave my sight until I am sitting on the plane.

Once finally arriving to my seat, I carefully place my passport and ticket in my bag, and slide it underneath the seat in front of me. Once we take off, I lean forward pretending to myself I am only going to grab my novel. However, I sneak a peak to ensure the two essentials are where they are supposed to be.

Before we land, flight attendants pass out the ridiculous customs cards we are supposed to fill out to go through immigration. What a load of crap, and whatever becomes of those little cards we hand to the scary looking person behind the glass at passport control? And those people *are* scary looking. I think they are either trained to be scary or just so bored out of their minds they become scary.

After I fill out the paperwork, my passport goes back in

my hand, but my return ticket remains in the bag, and I check once again to ensure it is there.

After passport control and customs, my passport goes back into my bag with my sighted return ticket. Once on the bus to the rental car lot, I keep a sharp eye on my large bag in the baggage jail by the door and clutch my smaller bag in my hand. I have to sneak a peak because I may have dropped my passport rather than placing it back into my bag after customs.

"No, no, no! I know it is in there!" What harm is it to look, though; you are just on a bus? But I do not want to succumb to such craziness because I watched my hand place the damn thing in there and then zipped it up. Oh, but just think how relaxed you will be after you see it in there. "Okay, okay, so look," and I do and it is right where I put it.

After leaving the car-rental office, I place my passport in my bag and head to my car. I place my large bag in the trunk and my backpack up front with me and lay my passport on the seat with my return ticket.

Once I check into my hotel room, I unpack my big bag and am happy everything is as I packed it. My small bag remains packed, but I remove the return ticket and passport and place them between some shirts in the drawer. Should someone wish to break into my room and try to steal them, they will never think to look for them there.

Finally the trip is done, and, until the trip home, I will only obsess about such things as saving the world and everybody in it.

Since being on my OCD medication, I do not travel

nearly as much as I once did. I joke to people that I used to own Southeast Asia because I traveled so regularly from Singapore to Hong Kong and to all areas just outside and in between. Now driving on Hwy. 98 in northwest Florida is my main route. I have no use for passports or plane tickets. I hope one day to travel extensively again because I will be able to enjoy the trip of getting there so much more.

The Numbers Two, Three, Six and Seven

In my early stages of OCD, I became obsessed with being possessed by the devil. For a reason I do not remember, the numbers two and three became very important as to whether I loved the devil or not. I would say to myself, "If you tap yourself twice, then you love the devil. If you tap yourself three times, then you don't love the devil." Then I thought maybe I should rather say, "If you tap yourself twice, you don't love the devil. If you tap yourself three times, you do love the devil." Two or three taps – which one resulted in which?

Since not being sure which number resulted in which consequence, I had to refrain from ever using the numbers two or three in rituals to prevent a consequence. For instance, I could no longer shoot two or three birds at myself because that might possibly mean I love the devil. I could no longer tap myself two or three times, no longer take two or three steps, no longer slap myself two or three times, no longer do two or three cartwheels, no longer blink two or three times, no longer tap the top of a door two or three times, no longer dig my fingernail deep into my thumb two or three times nearly drawing blood, no longer shut my eyes for two or three seconds while driving down the highway, no longer circle my thumb painfully around its connecting joints two or three times, no longer hop on one foot two or three times.......

Two or three turned into other numbers that were off limits. Any number divisible by them became unusable, so prime numbers became very valuable. Outside of this important discovery, I have really never known what was so special about a prime number, but thank goodness for them as tools for saving the world. Without them, the world and its inhabitants would have been destroyed in the years since my birth.

For some reason, however, the number 100 was okay to use when it came to tapping, shooting birds, blinking, etc., for completing rituals. Maybe its because it is such a round number or because it is such a large number. It seemed to carry enough weight when repeatedly doing something that many times.

The other number that really seemed to cause me a lot of pain was the number 6. Being one of the numbers in the "sign of the beast," it also became an unforgiving number to use to prevent a consequence. Two, three and six or any product thereof was dangerous territory, and if any of those numbers were used, most likely the ritual would have to be repeated using a different number.

Since the number seven is a prime number, it was usually the smallest number available for repetitive actions.

The number five is also prime, but two + three = five, and that number was considered just too dangerous because of its makeup. In relation to seven, one of my favorite jingles to relieve myself of an obsession was the tune, "Shave and a haircut, six bits." The tune has seven notes, or seven syllables in my case because I do not know a thing about music.

However, even though the number of syllables is only seven, singing the tune one time, or tapping the tune once was not nearly enough, and I would have to say it at least seven times, or 100 or more if necessary. Over time, I have grown to hate that tune for what I have made it to be: a tune sung to save myself, someone else or the world. Since it is widely used in electronic media as a bumper at the end of a joke, punch lines are usually ruined for me.

Another attribute to the tune is that seven notes also is an uneven number of notes. With the number being uneven, while at the same time dealing with objects like floor tiles in an amount greater to or less than seven, the end of the tune, when giving each tile its own note, is guaranteed to end on a different tile. The neat part about it being a tune with an odd number of syllables is the beginning of the tune will always eventually end up back at the beginning floor tile. No matter how many floor tiles involved, as long as it is an uneven amount and not divisible by seven, I could end up back at the beginning tile no matter how long it took.

If you find all this very confusing, it is. Figuring it all out takes time, but saving the world is a very important job and shortcuts should not be taken when it needs to be done right.

The Right Hand
of the Father

In church, I often heard in songs and in readings of the privileged place to be at "the right hand of the Father." The way I understand it is you definitely want to end up on God's right side and not on His left. As written in Ephesians 1:15-23, *"God put this power (His great power) to work in Christ when He raised him from the dead and seated Him at the right hand in the heavenly places, far above every name that is named, not only in this age but also in the age to come."*

With that particular verse, being on the right side seems like a pretty powerful place. So whenever I obsessed over an object, whatever place my eyes should land last should be at the right side. For instance, if I had to look at a woman's breasts for a certain amount of time to prevent her from getting cancer, I would have to look at the right-side breast only or last.

With the seven-note tune aforementioned, I would have to ensure the last note ended on the right breast. The dangerous part about ending up on the right one is I must decide before beginning the ritual, which is the right breast. Would it be on her right side or the one that is on my right? This decision was never made before the ritual was completed, so I always had to repeat the ritual when the decision was made as to which breast was the correct one. Once I agreed with myself on the correct one, and once I correctly completed the ritual, one more woman had been saved from a deadly disease.

In the Ephesians verse, the right hand sounds like the best place to be, but why is the left hand the place you never want to be? As written in Matthew 25:31-46, *"When the Son of Man comes in His glory, and all the angels with Him, then He will sit on the throne of His glory. All the nations will be gathered before Him, and He will separate people one from another as a shepherd separates the sheep from the goats, and He will put the sheep at His right hand and the goats at the left. Then He will say to those at His right hand, 'Come, you that are blessed by my Father, inherit the kingdom prepared for you from the foundation of the world.' Then he will say to those at his left hand, 'You that are accursed, depart from me into the eternal fire prepared for the devil and his angels'."* (Poor goats.)

Since the Matthew verse spells quite clearly the disadvantages of being on the left side, consequences could never be prevented with rituals completed on the left side of any object. Therefore, under all possible circumstances, rituals had to finish on the right side. Should that not be possible considering angles, I would have to perform other rituals to make ending up on the left side okay.

A good example would be obsessing that all balls on a pool table end up on the right side. If the table is uneven and they all end up on the left side, another ritual would have to be preformed. But then again, which side of the table is truly the left side…? Figuring out this one is going to be trouble resulting in hair pulling and much anxiety.

Becoming a Missionary

Shortly after arriving in Singapore, I set out to find a place to live suitable for my bride-to-be and me. She was still in the USA, so I had tons of freedom in choosing something I liked. I settled on an old British Officer's home in a neighborhood full of what the locals call "Black and Whites." They were the homes of the British military during the colonial period. There were different levels of housing considering the rank of the officer. The house I chose would have been middle to high level, but not the highest. It had three bedrooms, a large parlor, dining room, kitchen, a beautiful backyard and a small house in the back for housing servants.

When my fiancé arrived, she did not think it such a good idea to live there. I don't know why other than the place was not air conditioned and so large that we had to share the rent with housemates. I don't know why she thought that so unusual for newlyweds to share a home with another couple and to live without air conditioning on an island just above the equator.

Oh, and did I mention the pythons in the attic? I had a

lot to learn, especially that a woman's expectations need not be screwed with when getting married.

She would have been shocked to discover what my latest obsession was, and how it was going to completely change her life. Not that marrying me, looking for a new job, and moving halfway around the world was enough.

I suddenly became obsessed with becoming a missionary. For whom for, I had no idea except that it would be to spread the Holy Word to natives in some jungle or remote village. I did no studying on becoming a missionary, had no idea what qualifications were needed, and had no education on the subject, but knew I had to become one. I obsessed that it was the only way of getting into heaven, and that was a good enough reason to blindside my new wife upon her arrival to Southeast Asia.

Since only just arriving in Singapore, I had no car yet and had to take the bus to work. I must have been the only white guy (locals referred to us as "red-headed devils") onboard and the only one not thinking about the day ahead or the night before. I can only remember swaying to the movement of the bus, staring at all the greenery that is Singapore, and how I was going to break it to my wife that we were going to become missionaries.

In my first few weeks at my new job, one of the ladies at the office asked me to join her for a game of golf. Living on such a small island in Southeast Asia, you do not turn down an invitation to play golf. There is so little room on the tiny island nation that the opportunity to play does not come very often.

With someone else paying for the round, I really did not have any choice but to say yes. It would probably be my only chance to ever play golf in such an unusual place.

We were partnered with none other than a huge American black man who ran missions. It had to be an omen! This match was definitely made for a purpose, other than giving locals something to laugh at: a small Singaporean woman playing golf with a blonde white guy and a huge black guy.

I became obsessed with this man's occupation of doing missions, and I asked every question possible on the subject. My golf game was ruined because of the information desired, and his probably was, too, from the questions I asked. The thing that must have puzzled him most were my questions with a religious angle and his missions had nothing to do with religion. He worked for the American Embassy and ran missions to other countries relating to international trade. No matter how many times I questioned his missions with a religious angle, he kept steering it back to trade. I thought by continuing my line of questioning, he would finally give me an answer with a religious angle and I could build on that and maybe get a job doing religious missionary work! If he had had a gun, I think he would have shot me.

I did visit him at the embassy once, and he was very nice to meet with me. By then, I had overcome my obsession and he gave me contacts at the Singapore American School where my wife would eventually work. However, if he had truly understood my obsession and the underlying meaning of my conversation with him on the golf course, I am sure he would have refused my visit at the embassy. This obsession could have proved to be the result of a lost opportunity for my new bride.

Having OCD presents the illusion of walking a fine line between life and death, opportunity and missed opportunity, and positive and negative outcomes. This is why controlling the obsessions is so important, and why the rituals are so important in preventing consequences related to the obsessions. Therefore, people with OCD probably spend half their waking moments performing rituals to keep from falling on the wrong side of that fine line that they alone have created.

My obsession was becoming a missionary, my ritual was to ask this embassy worker a false line of questioning and the consequence was my realization this guy knew nothing about religious mission work. It did not solve my obsession of becoming a missionary (time and other obsessions finally did that). Fortunately, though, the embassy worker did not throw me aside as a nutcase but respected me enough as an American to provide information leading to my wife's employment. In this case, I fell on the opportunity side of that fine line!

Now that I control my obsessions with pharmaceuticals, those fine lines are not created by my imagination, but by the environment in which I am currently a part. Landing on the correct side of the line is done now with carefully planned strategies and not with time-wasting rituals.

Sympathy for Breathers and Non-Breathers

My obsessive-compulsive disorder not only made me passionate for the safety of humans, but also for animals and objects having no life.

I first realized this while living in New Orleans. I was walking to my little township of Lakeview to do some shopping and noticed a little bird under a tree shrieking something awful. Apparently, it had fallen from its nest and was standing there on the sidewalk crying for its mother. I sat and watched hoping to God someone else would notice. I went through the steps of what needed to be done. First, I would go home and get a ladder and bring it to town, then scoop up the little bird, climb my ladder and place it back in the nest. Coming back the next morning, finding the mother had abandoned the baby, I would take the bird home and call the animal sanctuary asking what to do to save the bird. That is as far as the thought process went because someone else walked up to the bird and stooped down. I took off leaving them with the enormous responsibility, and felt guilty for the rest of the day thinking I could have helped one of God's little creatures.

A few years later, I did all of that minus the ladder. I found a seagull on the beach with a broken wing. I went into the house and called the wildlife refuge and they told me to capture the bird and drop it off to them the next morning. I thought proudly, "What a wonderful thing I am doing for the animal kingdom." I searched out a box for me to imprison the gull, went out and captured it and left it in the garage overnight. The next morning I got up bright and early, and went to the garage to check on the bird. It was as dead as a doornail and stiff as a board, with its final hours having been spent in a lousy cardboard box when it could have been spent on the beach.

As a young child, I had a great maple tree in my backyard. It was a perfect climbing tree that could almost be ascended like a spiral staircase. One day, I was doing what any normal young boy would do climbing to the top of the tree and back. I inadvertently pulled a leaf off the tree as I probably did every time I played on it, but this time I became obsessed with this leaf. I had forced this leaf to separate from the tree prematurely of its natural demise in the fall. I felt terribly responsible for this, so I decided to not only save this leaf but to transform it into a great maple tree from which boys just like me could climb in years to come.

I brought the leaf into the house and told my mother I wanted to root it. She suggested putting it in a glass of water and placing it on the windowsill and probably never had a second thought about it. To me, however, this was a very important job because this leaf was going to die and, if not for me, it would be hanging gleefully from a branch high up on a tree.

After a day of waiting, nothing happened. After two days, the leaf looked sick and no roots were coming out. I realized this was not going to work, and this leaf was taking too much of my time and worry. So, I took the leaf out of the glass and took it outside. I ripped it in two and threw it into the yard. I was guilt stricken and must have been severely. Otherwise, who else would remember this insignificant boyhood experience? As written earlier in this book, as someone with OCD, I never forget anything, especially a negative experience.

Some thirty years later, another major incident took its toll on my time. In Gulf Breeze, FL, behind what was formerly the Bruno's grocery store was a number of cats. The season happened to have been winter, and I commonly used the trucking area behind the grocery store as a short cut to the post office. There were a number of dumpsters back there, so naturally there were cats. They were either feral cats or domestic cats looking for a mate or an extra bite to eat. We were having an unusually cold spell that winter and it was dipping down into the teens, so radio stations were making the usual announcements to drip your faucets, empty your hoses, look after aging neighbors and "FOR GOD'S SAKE, BRING IN YOUR PETS!"

I began to obsess about those cats and thought if they were not rescued, they were going to freeze to death. I told myself the reasons why they would be okay without my help: 1) They are wild animals, and they know how to take care of themselves; 2) They are pets from the houses behind the grocery store, and they will go home when gets too cold; 3) They could be sick and not well enough to bring into my home; 4) They have cats around them who are of their family and would not want to be broken up; 5) My cat, Bugsy, would be very upset if I allowed another cat into the house.

I thought about all of these reasons, but none could overcome the thought that if I did not go pick up these cats they would be dead by tomorrow. I fought my reasoning all the way home and into the living room. Alone with my thoughts, I knew time was of the essence. Nighttime was not far off, and it would soon be too dark to find them in that back alley. No ritual could save me from this obsession. There was nothing I could do to save those cats except to drive back to the store and pick them up.

I fought this obsession with mighty effort with my head in my hands and my fingers pulling at my hair. The time slowly went by, and by the grace of God and his creation of a rotating earth, the sun finally gave way to darkness.

The Uncomfortable, Lifeless Object

Not being completely sure how or when this obsession started, I began feeling sorry for objects having no nervous systems. Through OCD, I fooled myself into believing material objects had feelings.

One place it may have begun was with something as

simple as a tennis shoe. After all, a tennis shoe does have a tongue, and since objects may be looked at from different perspectives, a shoe is brought to life when it is looked at as a living creature. Without a foot in the shoe, it looks like it is screaming. Until a foot is inside, the shoe continues to scream. I found it difficult sometimes deciding which shoe to wear, because I felt sorry for the other ones who were going to be left in the closet screaming all day. When throwing a pair of shoes away, I always tie them together and place them in a plastic grocery bag. I never want them to become separated because I always feel sorry for single shoes lying on the side of the road. You almost never see a pair, just one, and it is usually lying on its side with its laces untied and its tongue hanging out. What happened to its mate? If only they had been tied together, they could keep each other company as they rot away.

When my family gathered once a year for the time-held tradition of decorating the Christmas tree (oh, it is supposed to be so much fun…it always is on TV), I would feel sorry for the decorations not chosen to hang from the tree that year. I would sneak around everyone and pick out the decorations set aside for later years, or for the trashcan for that matter, and place them on the back of the tree. Thankfully, my mother would usually stop me.

One year, during the annual Junior Service League charity attic sale, I bought a one-eyed purple and orange bulldog stuffed animal. It was probably the most hideous thing there (not that real bulldogs are very pretty), but I was afraid no one else would buy it, and it would end up in a garbage can somewhere. The bulldog would be so lonely and upset, and I could picture it whimpering. So with my hard-earned money, or weekly allowance, I purchased the stuffed animal and brought it into the safety of my home.

When my mother came into the house after her day working at the sale, she saw the dog. She said, "What is this thing doing back in the house?!" She was surprised, you see, because I bought that same dog at the sale last year, donated it to the sale this year, and then bought the ugly thing, again.

I also care about the physical comfort of material objects. Anything that has the least bit of elasticity has a normal position, unlike a pendulum or a piece of steel. For instance, if you slide a table across a floor, the legs of the table on one side may have bent slightly away from the direction of the slide, leaving them just a little off kilter. In my world of OCD, this means the table would be uncomfortable. To relieve the awkward feeling the table must have, each side of the table should be lifted so the legs fall naturally back into place. The carpet, too, could be stretched on one side of the slide, and buckled on the other. Lifting the legs helps that, too. I could not have the backing of carpet too stressed or bent, because that would be a very uncomfortable position for the carpet.

Another example could be a picture that was bowed after closing a drawer. In my world of OCD, the drawer would have to be opened to flatten out the picture into its original shape. I could also never pack something in a box that had to be bent (for instance a 12 inch flexible ruler in an 11 inch box). If something had to be bent to fit, it would be uncomfortable on its journey within the box and I would have to find a bigger box.

Even today, after taking many year's worth of medication, when I make up my child's bed, I have to make certain the stuffed animals don't bend over too far from the waist or have their heads bent backwards or too far forwards. I think what it would feel like to sit uncomfortably all day like that, and how painful it could become. The stuffed animal has no means by which to change its position, so I make sure it is left in a comfortable position before I leave the room.

Three Major Things

During most of my life, I heard people say the following things regarding my active lifestyle:

1. He is so hyperactive.
2. He could have fun in a closet.
3. He is full of energy.
4. He is the most fun person to be around.

Fitting every description, I am glad to have fooled almost everyone who was ever around me. Although I am not full of energy, or hyperactive, and I could never have fun in a closet. However, I *am* fun to be around.

In my early twenties, as with most people that age who are not married, I hung around a group of people freshly out of college who were at their first jobs or looking for one, freshly married or looking for a spouse, and typically having a good time doing both. Weekends and weeknights were spent footloose and worry-free with no real responsibilities to hold us back. Beginning salaries of $30,000 were more than enough to cover rent, groceries, a couple vacations and beer. The company car, gas card and car phone, of course, were great bonuses.

Fortunately for me, these years were spent in the warm climates of Sydney, Australia and Pensacola, FL. There was a lot outside of work that had to be done, and by God, I was going to do it. Not out of want, but because of obsessions.

While in Sydney, I developed the obsession of doing at least three major things a day on weekends. These activities may have included any combination of the following:

- Playing golf (golf was cheap in Australia)
- Flying kites
- Bodysurfing
- Beach-cliff climbing
- Sailing (I used to hitch a ride at the local sailing club with a heavy-drinking captain named "Jack.")
- Riding my bike
- Throwing the Frisbee or Aerobie
- Playing touch football (footie)
- Hiking
- Scuba diving
- Waterskiing

After all of that, I would go out to the pubs and attempt to impress the ladies. I could not wait to get to work on

Monday so I could rest.

Looking back, I can't believe all that I did while living in Sydney. Fortunately for me, I lived in a flat with many people my age and all of who became my friends. You could say I had an enormous supporting cast of characters who could rotate in and out of my activities. As if I was an alcoholic, these people were my enablers.

Puzzling as it was to many of them, and painful as it was for me, I would be having a great time doing one activity and all of a sudden make an exit. I had to get to my next major activity.

For Australians, this was very unusual behavior because of their laid-back culture. After they complete a task, they would usually be off to the pub for a beer and relax the rest of the day. Not me, though. I would leave that group and head back to the flat to ready myself for the next adventure. I would knock on the doors of those who may have slept through the day's first activity and get them to participate with me in the next. Sometimes it was hard, and sometimes it was easy, but I usually managed a supporting cast.

Once the second major venture was completed, I would move to the next leaving my second shift of friends behind. Sometimes, some of my friends would follow or I could find others to join me. At other times, I would be left alone and have to complete the third activity on my own. That was when this obsession brought me sorrow, because abruptly leaving something entertaining with friends whom I loved only to complete the third major thing alone was very depressing. But the day would not be complete without the final activity, and it had to be done!

Little did I know at the time, but I held a group of about 20 people together during my two years at the flat by cooking them breakfasts, organizing day trips, nights out and spontaneous events. When I came back to the USA, I learned the whole colony had fallen apart. Their cruise director had abandoned them.

After being there two years, I had seen and done more than most of my friends there had done their entire lives. It almost killed me, but I dove the Great Barrier Reef, skied the Snowy Mountains and the South Island of New Zealand, sailed Sydney Harbor and the Whitsunday Islands, walked the Salt Lakes of South Australia, explored the Coober Pedy opal mines, climbed and walked around Uluru (Ayer's Rock) and the Olgas, hiked the Blue Mountains, visited the museums and toured the parliament buildings of Canberra, attended performances at the Sydney Opera House, drove the Ocean Road where the Twelve Apostles lay just off shore, attended two Grand Finals (equivalent to our Super Bowls) in the sports of Rugby League and Australian Rules Football and even became a godfather to a boy in Queensland.

My OCD in Australia never allowed me to relax, which may have, in the end, not been such a bad thing. My doing three major things a day also influenced a publicity marketing piece for the Nova Scotia tourism council. When I lived in Singapore, one of my roommates returned home to Canada to work as a graphic designer, and she designed a tourism piece based upon my ritual promoting that visitors to Nova Scotia could do three major things a day while on vacation.

My latter years of lack of responsibility came once I returned to the United States. I again sought out a similar cast of characters to support my habit of three major things a day. Fortunately for me, I had a beach house in Florida at my disposal. Anyone with a beach house is bound to have plenty of friends.

I would have all three of my boats (a motorboat, a catamaran and a 22 ft. Catalina) rigged and in the water. I would ready my kites, water skis, floats, Frisbees and other beach toys for all to enjoy. All of this would take me hours, and done not because I wanted to, but because I had to. At the end of the day, others went to bed relaxed and smiling. I went to bed exhausted and miserable.

I now live permanently in Pensacola, FL. I still have my boats (minus the Catalina, but plus a Sunfish) and many other beach toys. My boats sometime sit idle for months at a time, and cutting vines away from their beached hulls is something I have to do. I am able to sit under a beach umbrella and, with no guilt, look at them unrigged and lifeless. Many of my beach toys are socked away in a closet, and if I have time to play with them, I will get them. I am much happier now enjoying my things when I want to, taking my time with enjoyable experiences, and enjoying the presence of friends without having to abandon them for another activity.

Formosan Termites, Squirrels
and
a Gas Furnace

In New Orleans, LA, some experts believe the entire French Quarter is home to one huge Formosan termite nest with a multitude of queens living in an enormous network of tunnels throughout the historical rotten wood.

On certain spring nights in the Crescent City, termites fly in swarms around streetlights, spotlights and floodlights. Sporting events become gruesome nightmares with nasty little creatures falling on cringing spectators and participants. If you have a lot of hair, be prepared to pick wood-destroying insects from your roots before heading to bed.

During the nights of the swarms, the streets were dark and deserted. Residents who had any sense turned off all their lights and used flashlights to find their way around the house. Even light from TVs and computer monitors attract the nasty creatures. Neighborhoods take on the semblance of a blacked-out British town preparing for an air raid during the

Luftwaffe's Blitzkrieg in World War II.

After the termites frantically search an hour or so for termite mates under the lights, the swarms disappear. The termites have landed, dropped their wings, and begin the ritual of reproducing or colonizing. Should they fail to colonize with their new mates, they will be dead the next morning.

On one such evening, unaware of a coming swarm, my wife and I went out to eat. We left before sundown and came back after the swarms had disappeared. As usual, before leaving the house, I had illuminated the light in the attic to make attractive the dormer above the front door. The termites had found our light, and our house was full of wingless termites engaging in sex.

They were crawling into the living area from the attic by way of a space between the crown moulding and the ceiling. There must have been thousands in the attic.

We stayed up killing as many as we could, and went to bed when they seemed to have stopped creeping in. The next morning we awoke in our Indonesian four-poster bed with the duvet covered in dead termites.

No husband in the world could let his wife go through the horror of that again. So with a caulk gun in hand, I crawled up into our attic and began sealing off any crack I could find.

Our home was located in the Lakeview area north of the city. It was built in 1920, and was not airtight. Fortunately, it was only 1,200 square feet. The attic was full of old insulation, dust, probably a few dead bodies, termite wings and a gas furnace. Whenever up there, I tried never to look too closely at what might be there.

Within the cracks between the roof and walls, I placed pieces of screen and then caulked over them. Behind the three dormer vents, only shielded from the elements with slanted wooden slats, I placed the same screen. Two problems were solved with the work on the dormers: termites and squirrels would be kept out. Little did I know at the time, but that screen behind the dormers would haunt me for years to come.

Fast-forward four years, and I get fired from my job. Without much to do, I look for a job and work on the house. Since my neighbors had told me they had seen squirrels regularly go in and out of my attic dormers, I decided to take a look. I found the screens had made perfect backstops for their nests. What a perfect setup for them with the screens making a nice foundation for their leaves, and a man-made roof over their heads protecting them from rain. When I was sure no squirrels or babies were in the nests, I removed the screens, trashed the leaves, and then replaced the screens.

After finding a job in Florida, I commuted back and forth from New Orleans for a year and a half. On the weekends, I would work on the house, take the garbage out and mow the lawn. On some occasions, my wife even noticed I had come home. Every now and then, I would clear out the nests in the attic to keep the contents from rotting and attracting termites, make sure there was enough airflow for the gas furnace, and replace the burned-out light bulb in the dormer window.

Finally, after 16 months of traveling back and forth, my wife decided having the trash taken out once a week was not enough, so she decided to move to Florida with me. We sold the house in New Orleans to a young doctor and bought a big house on a golf course in Gulf Breeze, FL. I loved my new home; it was modern, had plenty of insulation and was fairly airtight. I no longer had to worry about Formosan termites, or leaf-clogged dormers. I no longer had to, but I did.

We moved to Florida in July, when the termites were not swarming and there was no need for heating a house. I had essentially forgotten about my rotting leaves and suffocating gas furnace.

When winter arrived, bad thoughts began to creep into my head regarding the danger the young doctor was in. With the weather so cold he was bound to have the heater running full. Since gas fumes from the furnace had no escape from the "air-tight" environment I had created, it would most certainly filter through the same cracks between the moulding and the ceiling that the termites had used. The gas would then permeate the living area below and kill the unsuspecting sleeping doctor.

"No, no," I reasoned. The house inspector would surely have told the doctor about this possible danger when he bought the house. And besides, he probably goes up there periodically like I did.

No, he would never go up there. Only I was stupid enough to go into the hall closet, set up a shaky stepladder, and climb through that narrow hole in the ceiling into that nasty environment. That doctor was a bachelor, and what would he care if there were a couple of squirrels up there? Why would he care if the light bulb in the dormer window had burned out? He is definitely going to die from gas inhalation if I don't call him to let him know about the clogged vents.

I did not know his number, but of course knew the address so I decided to write him a letter, soon. I never wrote a letter and further suffered the obsession until the weather turned warm.

The seasons changed, and on another cold night, I would wish I had left him my carbon monoxide detector. This man was a doctor, though, and surely he was smart enough to get one of those. I must call him. I could look up his number on the Internet. "Oh no, I will not," my voice rings out while clinching my fists and leaning my head on a wall.

I am sure my former neighbors would have told him about the squirrels going in and out of the attic. He must already know and has had someone come in and remove the screens.

During the warmer months, I would forget about it again and all would be good. As soon as it got cold again, the obsession the doctor would die of gas inhalation would resurface. I would reason that the screens would have by now rusted or rotted enough under the weight of the nests and that airflow would have been restored, or that maybe I did not put screens on all of them and left the one in the back free and clear. "No, no, I am pretty sure they were all screened over, but not to worry they are definitely rotten by now and there is plenty of airflow for the furnace. He will be fine."

"No, he will be dead by February."

If he were to die, it would not be my fault, really. He

bought the house as is. On the release form, I was only asked to reveal lead paint and asbestos information. There was nothing on the form about known or unknown squirrels nests.

Another winter comes around, and he is surely going to perish this year. "No he is not. I am sure he must have bought his own gas alarm." Besides that, most smoke alarms have them included anyway. I should really call or write. But how foolish will I look doing that? The guy will think I am crazy, and he will tell the neighbors with whom I am still friends with that I am a loony. "Hey, now that is a good idea!" I should tell my old neighbors to tell him about the gas-fume-clogging nests in the attic and he will live on account of my heroics. Either that, or I can tell him myself next time I visit New Orleans.

I did eventually visit my old house again in New Orleans. My wife and I entered the house without even knocking. The door was ajar and the furniture inside was upside down. He had not changed the curtains and most of the fixtures were the same as well. The closets still had the good doctor's clothes hanging just as he had left them before he evacuated the premises. The culprit that had forced him out left its mark about eight feet up every wall, and it was not from a termite swarm or gas-filled air. The demise of that house was Hurricane Katrina and the breaking of the 17th Street Canal levee.

Shooting birds at myself, self inflicted pain, "Shave and a Haircut, Six Bits," tapping myself one hundred times, turning cartwheels, holding my eyes open for longer than I should without blinking, or any other ritual did not put an end to my obsessing over someone dying because of not revealing a flaw when selling my home. This obsession was overcome by a great flood of which displaced and killed many people. Thank you God that I could not think of anything I could have done to cause that flood.

Church

Hymnbooks and prayer books offer really fun games at church. As an Episcopalian, the congregation does a lot of sitting, kneeling and standing up, and that is good for someone with OCD – always some action. When the preacher and the congregation read together, I had to keep up with every word. If I missed a word, or read over a word or got one wrong, I would have to go back and re-read it as the congregation moved on. I would sometimes fall behind a line or paragraph but have to keep reading aloud until I caught up. It is kind of like starting your applause after everybody else and stopping your clapping after everyone else is finished, just so you get in the same amount of applause as everyone else.

The singing was the same story; I would have to play catch-up when falling behind. Of course I did this up quietly, but it was quite uncomfortable when the rest of the congregation had already moved to the kneeling position while I was still standing trying to complete a verse. What finally saved me from this game is the fact that I am a terrible singer, and my wife just told me to quit even trying to participate in singing hymns. I may attempt to make a joyful noise unto the

Lord, but my wife will not be of any witness to it.

Church was a pretty difficult place when OCD came into play. Surrounded by such holiness, the OCD-possessed mind usually pushes evil thoughts into the head. Sometimes I felt God was no match for my thoughts, and He could not heal me of such an awful affliction. I would pray like mad at church that He would save me. I sought one-on-one prayers with a priest and together we asked God to make the obsessions go away. Following each service, one of the priests would stand by the entrance way to a small chapel at the front of the church as though in wait for a victim to come forth. This particular Sunday, the priest was a lady. She and I walked together up the aisle of the miniature church, with the stain-glass windows depicting Jesus along on our right, the Altar to the front and little post office boxes in the rear containing remnants of the dead. The priest walked around the railing in front of the kneeler, turned to face me and asked me the subject of my prayer. I replied saying I wanted God to make my obsessions go away. I kneeled and she placed her hand on my head and prayed as if she new exactly what I meant. She asked God to rid me of my obsessions, that they were so difficult for us to live with and it was so difficult for us to rid ourselves of destructive thoughts.

Oh how I wish the prayer session had concluded as in the Gospels where Jesus touches demonic subjects and the demons suddenly make a permanent exit from the body. No such luck for me, but I was surprised at how the priest had been so compassionate and seemed to know exactly the excruciating pain I was experiencing.

As an acolyte in my younger years, my church installed a new pipe system for the organ. The rector had been talking about it for months, and the church was certainly crowded for the grand unveiling. As the procession approached the Altar, I remember looking at the pipes instead of looking ahead, because I had seen in movies where people look in awe at a beautiful sight. I said to myself, as if I was really impressed, "Oh my, oh my!"

In the interest of a desire to be impressed, thinking I was supposed to be, I could have tripped over something causing the torchbearers to fall to the floor, dropping their candles, catching fire to the carpet and burning the whole place down. Truth is, I hate organs and prefer attending services when the pipes don't make a sound because no one is there to tend to the keys.

What is an organ anyway? Is it a cheap imitation of a symphony? I don't know, but if anyone really thinks the horn sounds it makes sounds like a horn, they must have a great imagination.

Every time I go to that church and walk up to the Altar for communion, I cringe at the lying I did to myself on that day. I still repeat to myself, "Oh my, oh my!"

One of my most memorable OCD church experiences was at a wedding, and I can still picture it as if it was yesterday. During the wedding of one of my father's business partner's daughters, I was sitting at the perfect position by the aisle where the bride was to march to the Altar. As her pretty smile lit the way toward her husband-to-be, I became obsessed with stepping on the flowing train behind her. As she passed, I wanted to put my foot out into the aisle and wedge the train between the carpet and the bottom of my shoe. The train would come off with a rip and land on the floor. The beaming smile would have disappeared, and a red-faced bride would have left the church in tears.

Thankfully, none of this happened, the bride got safely by me and I performed some other ritual so that she could. She should have thanked me for thinking of an alternative ritual, but she never did.

Even the act of going to church was an obsession. Sometimes, I really wanted to attend, and other times I had to attend. While in college, I would go to the local Episcopal Church and hope I would be too late to join the worship, and therefore I could not to attend. While living in Sydney, Australia, there was an Anglican Church right across the street from my flat, and I would go at least once every two weeks to the early service. The preacher was extremely boring and the service was fairly drab, but I made myself go anyway. It was not that big of a deal considering none of my friends were even up yet and still asleep when I returned.

While visiting nearby Manly Beach one day, I discovered a nicer church with a younger crowd. It was very vibrant and people were very kind and welcoming, so I decided to attend that church. The problem was that church was a 30-minute drive from my flat, and, with evening services, I would miss spending time with my friends who had really become my family.

I would be out playing with my flatmates on a Sunday afternoon, and then obsess about going to church. I tried not to look at my watch and hoped time would pass before noticing how late it was. My time with these people was very limited, because I was heading back to the United States soon.

Towards the end of my time in Sydney, I was sitting in the flat with my friends, and I obsessed to the point of creating an enormous amount of guilt upon myself for not welcoming the gift of worship at the church. I know now, and really knew then, that God's gift was in that room with me, and I should have spent every last second with my soon-to-be long-distance friends. The obsession, however, was too strong and I left so to complete the ritual. The OCD consequence of me not completing the ritual was making bad decisions regarding my future employment. The real consequence was loosing precious last moments with my friends, some of whom I have not seen since.

Following my marriage, and our subsequent move to Singapore, I continued my obsession there, too. I attended another Anglican Church, and it was really cool. It had a large covered area with no walls, but the décor was as any indoor church would be. Most who attended were ex-patriots, mostly from the US, UK, Canada and Australia. I enjoyed going to the services before my wife arrived, because Singapore was a fairly boring place and there was not much going on Sunday mornings anyway.

When my wife did arrive, however, the obsession struck

again. I was a newlywed, and I insisted we go to church. There were other things we could have done as a couple, and we would have been much happier doing them instead.

I am certainly not knocking the church, but it is so much more enjoyable to attend when you actually desire to worship rather than attend to satisfy an obsession. Out of all of my obsessions, I think this one was the most painful because I felt guilty making myself go, I felt guilty while I was there, and I felt guilty for the time I spent away from something more enjoyable. Obsessions rob a person of life, and God gave me life. I was wasting it by putting forth a fake desire to worship Him when I truly was only satisfying an obsession.

In the end, however, I showed friends who did not attend church, that it was okay to go and give thanks for His many blessings. I also prayed to God at every church service that He would free me of my obsessions, and He eventually did after I waited so very long for His help. I often wondered where He was the whole time I was asking Him to help me. I did eventually find out where He was, and that the act of my waiting for His help was a complete waste of time.

Waiting for God

When I was fourteen years old, I began to experience something that was not normal. I can remember the exact moment it began, and I can't even remember whom the first girl was that I kissed. It was with one of two girls, but I can't remember which one it was. I certainly hope she doesn't remember that first kiss either.

For me to remember the exact moment this whole mental thing started shows it was a major, life-changing experience.

It was a summer day, and I was watching a baseball game. All of a sudden my mind began taking a great interest in the pitcher-catcher sequence. The actions and the order in which they occurred did not concur with what my brain had imagined, and I could not satisfy the demands made on me by my brain. All of a sudden I found myself counting to 30 before each pitch, or depending on the pitcher to grab his crotch before the catcher gave a signal, or wanting the hitter to spit at least twice before entering the batter's box. If any of these demands were not met, I found myself having to find some other situation to make up for the last unsatisfied demand such as having the pitcher make at least two of those useless throws to first base in an attempt to pick off the first-base runner. The two throws had to be consecutive and not spread out in the pitching sequence.

Sometimes the announcers came into play, and I demanded certain things for them to say, like the pitch count, or "Have a look at that youngster in the stands." Then there was the organ, that stupid organ playing the "Charge!" trumpet call. How stupid is that? The only charge in baseball is when a hitter charges the mound, and that is not even really part of the game. Who thought it would be a good idea to have an organ at a baseball game? I guess it was a good idea because there is one at almost every stadium (excuse me, ballpark) to ensure it annoys someone. It is almost as annoying as "Batter, batter, batter, swing!"

Just maybe it was the act of watching a baseball game that put me over the edge and changed my life forever. Like a little league right fielder becoming a slave to the most boring position, I became a slave to these unfamiliar demands.

It was as if another person had taken up residence inside of my head. I tried to reason with myself, turned off the game and worried about what was happening to me. I went out into the backyard and put my head in my hands and rubbed my eyes. I had changed my environment, but my brain suddenly made new demands on me having nothing to do with audio or video. The TV had been turned off, but to my horror I realized turning off the TV did not stop these thoughts. They kept coming to me at the speed of light, and I prayed the thoughts would subside with time.

The thoughts would not go away, and I did not tell anyone about them. Should there have been a pain in my side or an open wound, my mother or father would have been the first to know about it. They would have taken me to the doctor and demanded a diagnosis. Prescriptions or procedures would have put me on the road to recovery.

However, this was a problem that was not visible and very hard to explain. It would have been embarrassing to discuss because it seemed so stupid, and it could not be physically observed. It was like a UFO sighting, and no one would believe me if I told them. Even in the 70's television show, "Project UFO," I remember it usually ended with the Air Force investigators telling the UFO witnesses, "We can't prove that you did see it, but we can't prove that you didn't." I was afraid my diagnosis would be similar, so I just kept quiet and kept on suffering.

The Ugly Years and God

Being 13 and 14-years old was tough. I refer to those ages as the ugly years, because hair starts to get greasy, acne creeps along, braces go onto the teeth, feet get big, whiskers start growing, grades start going downhill, parents start talking responsibility, blah, blah, blah.

Funny how all of this ugliness sets in at about the same time our mind decides it is time to start taking an interest in the opposite sex. Oh, I had seen dirty magazines and lusted over Charlie's Angels, but up to this point in my life I had no intention of actually asking a girl on a date (albeit to the seventh-grade dance at the school gym, and this girl was in the sixth grade and not Farrah Fawcett Majors). "Hi my name is Donald, and would like to go to a dance with me and my zit and new braces." Amazingly she said, "Yes." I did not speak with her again until the dance five days later.

God was also becoming part of my life, and when I turned seventeen it occurred to me that I actually needed Him and should really get to know Him. I did not know any of my jobs until I worked them, I did not know my wife until I married her and I didn't know God until I got into a heated, albeit one-sided, conversation with Him.

One day, I had it out with God about a very serious matter. I was screaming at Him and berating Him for not lending a helping hand. It was on that day I came to grudgingly understand that He, in fact, is the one in charge and the one who decides the timing of His assistance.

I met with my preacher regarding this incident and he asked me how I was praying. I told him I was praying for God to strengthen someone, so they may see the light. He looked at me and said, "You do not need to ask God to give this person strength. This person has plenty of strength. You need to be straight with God, and you need to pray for *your* strength."

The message I got was not to beat around the bush when I pray. God is very busy and does not have time for our earthly guessing games. He has things like war, famine and natural disasters to deal with, so He needs to know what you need, so in turn you will know what you need. If you are true to God in your prayer to Him, you will be true to yourself.

There is a cartoon by Gary Larson, author of the "Far Side," depicting two men playing on a TV trivia game show. God is behind one lectern, and He is about 8 feet tall with long white hair and a beard and wearing flowing robes. His score is 1,151,430. His competition is a typical "Far Side" nerd behind a lectern with a score reading, "ZERO."

Then there is the line in our prayer book read every Sunday in my church reading, "From whom no secrets are hid." The "whom" is referring to the Almighty.

The point is, God already knows our problems, and He made us in His image. But He did not make us perfect. If He did, what kind of challenging life would we, or He have? He did give us, however, problem solving ability, and for some reason we don't use it a whole lot on ourselves because of a few reasons:

1. We don't want to admit we have a problem.
2. We think the problem will go away.
3. If we admit we have a problem, we have to tell someone else about it in order to get help.
4. We may be too stupid to know we have a problem, and in some cases that may not be such a bad thing.

As I grew older, entered high school, got my driver's license and began dating, thoughts uncontrollable to me began consuming my everyday activities.

I took these mind games to college, the fraternity, spring breaks, graduation, to my job in Australia, engagement, marriage, my job in Singapore, unemployment, New Orleans, Pensacola and to a weekend in Apalachicola, FL.

My life was completely consumed by something I had no idea could be diagnosed and controlled, and yet no one knew of my problem: not my parents, sister, friends, teachers, coaches or my wife. I am sure, with my wife looking back on our marriage, she has a better understanding of some of the things I did: needlessly working on an outboard motor the day before leaving for Singapore (I paid little attention to her and was not going to see her for months), getting her up at the crack of dawn on our honeymoon insisting we see all the sights of Paris, and almost killing myself swimming to an island in Malaysia. It all *had* to be done.

My family and friends knew I was suffering from some sort of disorder when I, an Auburn graduate, married an Alabama graduate. I prayed to God he would save me from this agony, but nothing happened. (Of course not the agony of being married to an Alabama graduate. I am learning little by little, everyday, to live with that.)

Crossing Over From the Dark Side

A light at the end of a tunnel is what you see when you are almost there. I never could see the light at the end of my tunnel because of the complete darkness of my disorder. Everywhere I turned, there was no escape from my mental illness. Only temporary escapes from my obsessions through rituals offered short relief until they were deemed useless by the next obsession. My living hell had to come to an end. I had to see someone, tell someone what was happening to me. But whom would I see, and what would I tell them?

Put Your Hands on the Radio

Somewhere along the way, I understood my problem to be the result of a chemical imbalance in the brain. Whenever I had really bad days (some seemed to be worse than others), I would say to myself, "Boy, the chemicals in my brain are really out of whack today!" I actually said this to make myself feel better about my situation. It was more like a lie giving me false comfort that better days lay ahead.

The problem continued to grow worse. From the moment I woke up in the morning to the moment I went to bed, this lingering disorder shadowed my every move.

Nothing got by me. I noticed everything, remembered everything, pondered every thought and never had to write anything down. I wished for real problems to occur, so I could concentrate on those rather than the silly ones made up in my obsessive mind. My mind began to include the silly games in my dreams. I was in deep trouble, and I was still waiting for God.

Over 2,000 years ago, God sent a Jew into the world to save us all. You will read on bumper stickers crediting a Jewish carpenter as the Christian savior. Well, a Jewish-radio-talk-show host saved my life.

I was in Navarre, FL on October 24, 2002, with my radio tuned to "The Dennis Prager Show." He had a guest, Dr. Jeffery Schwartz, on the show and they were speaking of his book, *The Mind and the Brain*. It was a book detailing the problem I had and people were calling in talking about the disorder I was living with. The problem had a name, and it was Obsessive Compulsive Disorder – OCD. Calls came in from all over the country from people having various obsessions including one woman who would picture herself stabbing her own daughter with a kitchen knife. She explained she was controlling these thoughts with drug treatments. Others called in and said they were using therapy. The difference between those people and me was they were actually doing something about their problem.

I did, however, get the name of what the disorder was, and now I was able tell God what it was, and He could help me. I thought He needed *my* diagnosis so He could divinely prescribe the right medicine. I began praying to God to help me specifically overcome my OCD. Another year went by, and He still did not help.

God had to have been frustrated with me at this point. He has spent years making humans self-sufficient. I guess He felt He no longer had to perform such miracles as having bread rain from the sky. That is what I was hoping would happen – that some cure would just all of a sudden appear.

Either I did not have the courage to seek help from His worldly creations, or I just wasn't smart enough to look in the right places. He has given us doctors and prescription drugs, counselors, preachers, therapists, libraries and the Internet. The answer to my problem was somewhere within modern miracles. If the Bible were written today, miracles would not be in the form of bread or the parting of seas, but in the form of updated software, a recharged car battery, a backup of accidentally deleted files, a medical procedure, a new set of house keys that had been lost or the safe landing of an impaired jet.

I could still not see the light and was waiting for bread to fall from the sky. Life was no longer fun. Everything I did was not because I wanted to do it, but because I had to do it. With OCD, an obsession is never satisfied and the compulsions or rituals continue throughout every waking hour. The problem led to artificial worrying, mouth ulcers, anxiety and, finally, guilt.

I was spending too much time in my life dealing with things that did not matter. I could not do anything for enjoyment. I could not relax and vacations were hard to enjoy. Sailing, tennis and flying kites were not relaxing. I had trouble reading books and watching movies.

After having reached the age of 37, twenty-three years after this whole mess began I finally heard God's answer to me in the form of a lie. It was a harmless lie to my wife about a grocery store visit. (I told her I visited a shop down the street, but I actually drove to another store 30 miles away to make sure I had not caused a wreck in that area earlier in the day.) I realized at that time my lies covering my future obsessions could become worse and even threaten my marriage. This particular lie followed a weekend trip to Apalachicola, and we spoke for the first time after 10 years of marriage about something that was killing me. I was on the way to recovery.

The next day my father came over for some unexpected reason, got what he needed, and prepared to leave. I stopped him and told him I needed to talk to him about something. We sat down on the back porch of my home, and I revealed to him I had a problem. I cried like a baby while looking at his concerned face and reassured him that it was not drugs or alcohol. As those words came out of my mouth, the light at the end of the tunnel appeared, and I suddenly realized this was something I could defeat because it was not an addiction to a deadly substance.

Still having trouble explaining to him my issues, I sobbed, "I have saved the world from destruction so many times." He suggested I call my rector, and that was pretty much all the advice he had. I don't think he knew what else to say. He then told me about my sister who years ago had a disorder. He said she came to him with an article in a magazine about a girl with a disorder. After he read the article, he looked up at my sister with a "so" look on his face, and she replied to him, "That girl in the magazine is (metaphorically) me." He said the next day he took her to Atlanta for treatment. I guess he was either telling me I was not the only one in the family to be screwed up, or that my problem could be overcome as her problems were overcome.

The next day my father called me and asked if I had called my preacher. I hadn't. After a week went by, he called again and asked if I had called. Nope. What I was waiting for, I do not know. Perhaps it was the thought of giving up my companion who had been by my side for so long. I began to feel like an alcoholic who suddenly decided on his own that admission was enough and I could handle it from here, with a half-empty bottle beside me.

I finally called my preacher and told him, and he referred me to a psychologist. After speaking with the psychologist and describing to him some of my obsessions and rituals, he said I needed drugs and not therapy. He then referred me to a psychiatrist. I called the psychiatrist's office, and the receptionist asked what I wanted to discuss with the doctor. I told her I would save the details for him, but she insisted I had to tell her before she could make the appointment. For the first time I was telling a perfect stranger (besides the professional psychologist) of my problem. From that point on, the more people I told about my mental illness, the easier it got, and I felt for the first time in forever the wind at my back.

Visiting my Psychiatrist's Office

During my first appointment, the good psychiatrist asked me the typical questions you would expect from a shrink: "How is your sex life? Do you hate your parents? Have you thought about suicide?"

I said I thought about suicide once, but if I had to take this problem with me to the afterlife, I would prefer not even going.

My psychiatrist's office was not as I expected it would be, and he was neither Frazier Crane nor Bob Newhart. He did not request I lay on a couch and there was no homey feel about the office. There were no dark paneled walls and attractive bookcases or expensive lamps on nice coffee tables. The carpeting was not plush and my fancy drink was only bottled water. The office was much like an attorney's office with three-ringed binders and professional books lined on plain looking shelves, commercial-industrial carpet, tiled ceilings and humming florescent lighting.

My first meeting was a one-hour appointment. Every minute was very stressful, and I was very nervous. I felt really stupid telling him about my episodes with OCD and anxiety attacks. But unlike the "twinkling eye" look Santa Clause gave the character in "'Twas the Night Before Christmas," my doctor gave me the look that this confession was no different than many others he had already heard from other patients.

The clock could not move slow enough, because the more I spoke about my experiences, the more I had to say. After the hour was up, I was exhausted and out $180.00.

The good doctor started me off with 50 milligrams a day of Zoloft. He had a bunch of sample bottles holding just a few pills apiece, and we made another appointment two weeks out. After taking the first little pill, I noticed a small difference, but they also made me feel sick. I lay on the couch for some time after swallowing the first one and waited for the mind alteration to begin.

After two weeks on the pill-a-day program, they had stopped making me feel sick, and I went back to the doctor for a $135.00, forty-five minute appointment. I told him I could tell a difference in that my obsessions were still overwhelming but the necessity of my having to perform rituals had eased up just a fraction. So he gave me another bag full of barely filled bottles, told me to take two pills a day, and we set an appointment for four weeks out.

Taking 100mgs of Zoloft a day did not make me feel physically different and did not have much more of an affect than did the 50mgs. My obsessions were still extreme, and I still had to perform rituals. What I found amazing about my unrelenting condition is that I had spoken to a professional about my obsessions and rituals in agonizing detail to no avail.

I would even witness my doctor shaking his head in disbelief at some of my OCD stories. He looked at me one day and said, "You are the perfect example of someone with OCD." He was so impressed with my ritual of my foot having to hit the floor before the door closed behind me that he had me recreate the sequence in his office.

I thought after someone had heard my stories, and of me hearing myself tell the stories to a willing listener, I would somehow be set free because of realizing the ridiculousness of it all. My doctor already knew, and I was beginning to understand, I was never going to be cured of OCD through therapy or medication. My sessions were only for the doctor to find the right medication and the right dosage of medication to temporarily, and on a daily basis, suppress the obsessions and to render rituals unnecessary.

My third appointment was a $95.00, 30-minute session. I arrived a few minutes early to make a list of my latest obsessions to discuss with the doctor because new ones were still making themselves available. Sometimes they were like dreams, though, and I had to think hard to recall just what the newest ones were. Following that session, we went up to 150mgs of Zoloft and samples were still available.

My next two appointments were also thirty minutes. I was happy with the 150mgs, and did not want to go to the max of 200mgs. My mind was altered enough and I was still questioning the possibility of damage to my brain, liver or whatever else as a result from taking these drugs. My doctor assured me the pills were not addictive and no long-term consequences should result from continuous ingestion. In the back of my mind, however, I could hear those 1-800-number lawyers advertising, "If you or someone you love has become ill from taking Zoloft, please call the number on your screen. You or your loved ones may be entitled to compensation for permanent brain and liver damage."

The next three appointments jumped back to $135.00, 45 minute sessions, because I was jumping back and fourth between 150 and 200mgs. At 150, almost all anxiety had disappeared except for the major issues of my causing the loss of a soldier in battle, the passport/terrorist obsession and the pizza incident.

Yes, the pizza incident. I have not written of it yet, so this is how it goes: It occurred after an Auburn football game where some friends and I helped a drunken fan to his car. He inadvertently, I am sure, gave us a $20 bill for helping. We hit a pizza place and left without paying because the waitress did not come to our table again, and the lady at the cash register yelled at us when we tried to pay at the counter. So we just walked out. I brought it up to one of my partners in crime twenty years later and experienced an anxiety unheard of for a seemingly harmless juvenile eat-and-run. For years I would add up what the cost of that pizza would be now with compounded interest. Even after a decade of treatment, I was not completely at ease until thirty years later when I did a drive-by of the restaurant's location and found that it was gone.

Since these three major issues still bothered me at the time, my doctor decided to keep me at the max of 200mgs.

Anything beyond that amount would not further its effectiveness.

As my appointments continued with my telling of OCD stories peppered with life saving rituals, anxiety, and shame, the good doctor made me realize having the disorder did have its advantages:

1. My magazines have been successful because of my obsession that everything must be spelled correctly, and ads, articles and points of reference must be to perfection.

2. During my weekends, I had to accomplish three major things a day. Some days I would sail, play nine holes of golf, and then ride my bike 20 miles. This was particularly effective while living overseas and especially in Australia. After two years, I had seen and done more than most of my Australian friends had done their entire lives.

3. My yard and my house were perfect. Now on the road to recovery, my wife noticed the house was not as clean as it used to be.

4. OCD also kept me out of trouble and helped to instill self-discipline. Anything less would have resulted in disastrous consequences: Drinking a beer and driving would have meant getting a DUI, having premarital sex would have resulted in a pregnancy or an STD, and a simple prank would surely have meant jail time. Well, I have not received a DUI, been in jail, caught an STD or

gotten anybody accidentally pregnant.

Growing up, my sister always called me "Goody Two-Shoes." It hurt because I knew there was an underlying reason for me not going out on a limb, but I did stay out of trouble.

At the tenth appointment, lightning struck. The good doctor had run out of Zoloft samples. I had to purchase those suckers and they ran $135.00 for one month. I never, in my life, spent that much on pills. I would though, and always would because that drug has saved my life. Even if I knew it would take 20 years off my life, I would take that loss for being able to live 20 happy years.

Now on the maximum dosage, obsessions do bubble up to the surface from time to time, and I have to perform very minor rituals. However, these rituals and obsessions are minor and completely manageable. The anxiety I feel during these post-medication attacks is very low and the obsessions are quickly forgotten and not dwelled upon. If I have an obsession about having to redo or perfect an action to prevent a consequence, I just move on, like walking away from a fight I know will have a useless outcome. The further I walk away, the less I feel the pull of the obsession and it quickly fades away.

I now visit my psychiatrist once every six months. I sit there in a chair across from his desk and try to think of something to say. This is my second doctor since my first has retired. With the first one, once my disorder was under control, we talked about college football for fifteen minutes, he filled out my prescription and I wrote him a check for $75. My new doctor is Columbian and does not care about college football. He asks me the same question every six months: "Do you feel your prescription is working?" I say, "Yes." Then he throws in how he is progressing in putting all his files into electronic form to meet government regulations, then looks at me for some kind of feedback while my mind is either somewhere in the Caribbean or replaying an Auburn football victory over Alabama. After stares are exchanged, he writes me a six-month prescription, and I write him a seventy-five dollar check.

The Last Word

As far as my problem is concerned, it is now under control, and I am the happiest I have been since I was fourteen-years old. Don't get me wrong, though. I had a great deal of fun during the rough years. Nothing could replace six years in college, four years overseas, and the first few years of marriage. However, I would have had a lot more fun had I just not waited for God, but listened to Him much earlier.

Every morning I take two little yellow pills (I call them my little Jesuses). Sometimes I forget, and my wife reminds me to take them if she notices me doing odd or repetitive actions. I always thank her for reminding me to take them, even if I already have done so. I don't at all consider her observations an insult, and I am happy someone is looking out for me.

Of the many gifts I have received from God regarding OCD, a financial one was when the patent of my "little Jesuses" finally expired allowing the sale of a generic. After my doctor ran out of samples, I was paying about $135 a month for a prescription. Once it went generic, the cost decreased to a little over $5 a month, back up to about $20 a month, and now, with a Sam's Club membership, it runs about $8 a month.

I love to talk about my problem and how I have been able to deal with it. I used to hope speaking engagements would become available so I could share my experiences but none have arisen since speaking at my church to a small group of people. In the church bulletin announcing my speech, the tagline under my picture read, "Donald Russell will be speaking of how he overcame a mental illness with God's help." Oh what my old girlfriends would have thought if they had read that bulletin.

Other speaking engagements never materialized, but, one day, I did get the opportunity to speak to hundreds of thousands of people. I was listening once again to "The Dennis Prager Show" on the radio. The subject of the day was "Do mental-health medications work?" Just as I heard him announce the topic at the top of the hour, I phoned the call screener and told her about the show I had listened to 14 years earlier. They put me through at the bottom of the hour. I was able to speak for about four minutes to the host about the disorder, the suffering endured for so many years, some examples of obsessions and rituals and of God finally coming to the rescue. Nothing would please me more than having my little contribution to the radio show encourage someone to seek out professional help for OCD or any other disorder, realizing that there is a cure out there, somewhere.

I also speak to a lot of people one-on-one. Sometimes the subject just comes up from overhearing people talk about their children or parents suffering a disorder or getting into intimate conversations with friends about daily problems. Being so confident to talk of my disorder, people begin to openly speak to me about their situation nervously, at first. They always whisper to me while I speak normal and openly. At times, people reveal to me things they have never told anyone else about their childhood or current situation. Once it just happened at a social gathering of tennis friends.

Another time, one of my clients asked me back to her office, and behind closed doors she tearfully told me of her extreme anxiety problems. I told her God had definitely brought us together that day, because my problems were as bad as hers, and I actually persuaded her to see a psychiatrist!

The greatest gift God gave to me was the decision to not let a disorder or problem bog me down and instead to do something about it. He taught me not to live with a problem that can be solved. Now I have a gift of being able to help others with similar problems, and hope to use that gift over and over again.

Ask God for help, and then listen and look around. Help will arrive or will already be there. The body cannot rest until the mind can. Have faith, don't sit idle and don't give up.

I wasted so much time waiting for God, because He was always there. I just didn't notice His presence until the day I revealed to my wife my disorder. He was sitting right there next to me, on the couch in my living room, pushing me to finally say the words to my wife that would lead to my healing: "Jenny, I have a problem."

Acknowledgements

I would like to thank the following people for helping me make this book possible: Michelle Kennedy Woodall for her photograph and creation of this gorgeous book cover; Kathy Lee Sumner, author of the novel *Captiva Island*, for pushing me to finally publish this book and for providing guidance in the publishing process; The Rev. Dr. Russell J. Levenson, Jr. of Saint Martin's Episcopal Church in Houston, TX for proofing my book from a spiritual perspective; Sara Daniel, broadcasting and PR specialist, for advising me on the order and flow of the book; Susan Anderson Nitterauer, author of *Cold Case in Ellyson*, who found many errors and marked the book up so viciously it almost hurt; Don, my father, and my mother Marilyn Russell, and my sister and brother-in-law, Kathy and Chris Dyleski for being the first to read the rough draft. Finally, I would like to thank my daughter Lauren, who at six-years old noticed page numbers missing in the final proof.

I would also like to thank those outside the writing process: My psychiatrists Dr. Mobley and Dr. Cruz of Pensacola, FL, and Dennis Prager, of the "Dennis Prager Show." By listening to his radio program, I came to understand my problem was not uncommon and could be treated.

I would also like to thank God!

About the Author

Donald E. Russell, Jr. sells advertising for tourist magazines in Northwest Florida. He is also the owner, publisher, editor, photographer, writer and distributor of those publications. He has previously sold carpet, raised flooring, work boots and peaches.

He graduated from Auburn University in 1989 with a Bachelor of Science Degree in Marketing, and attended the University of Florida School of Journalism in 1992 with a concentration on magazine journalism and radio broadcasting.

He has lived and worked in Australia, Singapore, the United Kingdom, Louisiana, Alabama, Florida and Georgia, and his life experiences, more than education, are the foundation of his knowledge.

He has felt the desire to help others in some fashion, and, after finally understanding his mental disorder, decided to spread the word that OCD can be controlled. Following a speech he gave to a church group about his disorder, he discovered that no one in the audience perceived him as crazy or unclean. Since then, his passion has been to tell others of what living with OCD is like and where to look for help.

Made in the USA
Columbia, SC
21 February 2021

33344228R00131